MCQs for the First FRCR

MCQs for the First FRCR

Dr Varut Vardhanabhuti MBBS BSc(Hon) DHMSA
Speciality Registrar, South West Peninsula Deanery, UK

Dr Julia James MBBS BSc(Hon) MRCS
Speciality Registrar, South West Peninsula Deanery, UK

Dr Rosemary Gray MBBS BSc(Hon)
Speciality Registrar, South West Peninsula Deanery, UK

Dr Rehaan Nensey MBBS MRCS
Speciality Registrar, South West Peninsula Deanery, UK

Dr W M Vivien Shuen BM MSc(SEM) MRCS
Speciality Registrar, South West Peninsula Deanery, UK

Dr Tishi Ninan MBBS MRCS
Speciality Registrar, South West Peninsula Deanery, UK

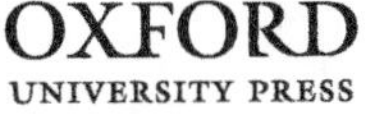
OXFORD
UNIVERSITY PRESS

OXFORD
UNIVERSITY PRESS

Great Clarendon Street, Oxford OX2 6DP
United Kingdom

Oxford University Press is a department of the University of Oxford. It furthers the University's objective of excellence in research, scholarship, and education by publishing worldwide. Oxford is a registered trade mark of Oxford University Press in the UK and in certain other countries

First published 2010
Reprinted 2012

British Library Cataloguing in Publication Data
Data available

Library of Congress Cataloging in Publication Data
Data available

ISBN 978-0-19-958402-4

Printed and bound by CPI Group (UK) Ltd, Croydon, CR0 4YY

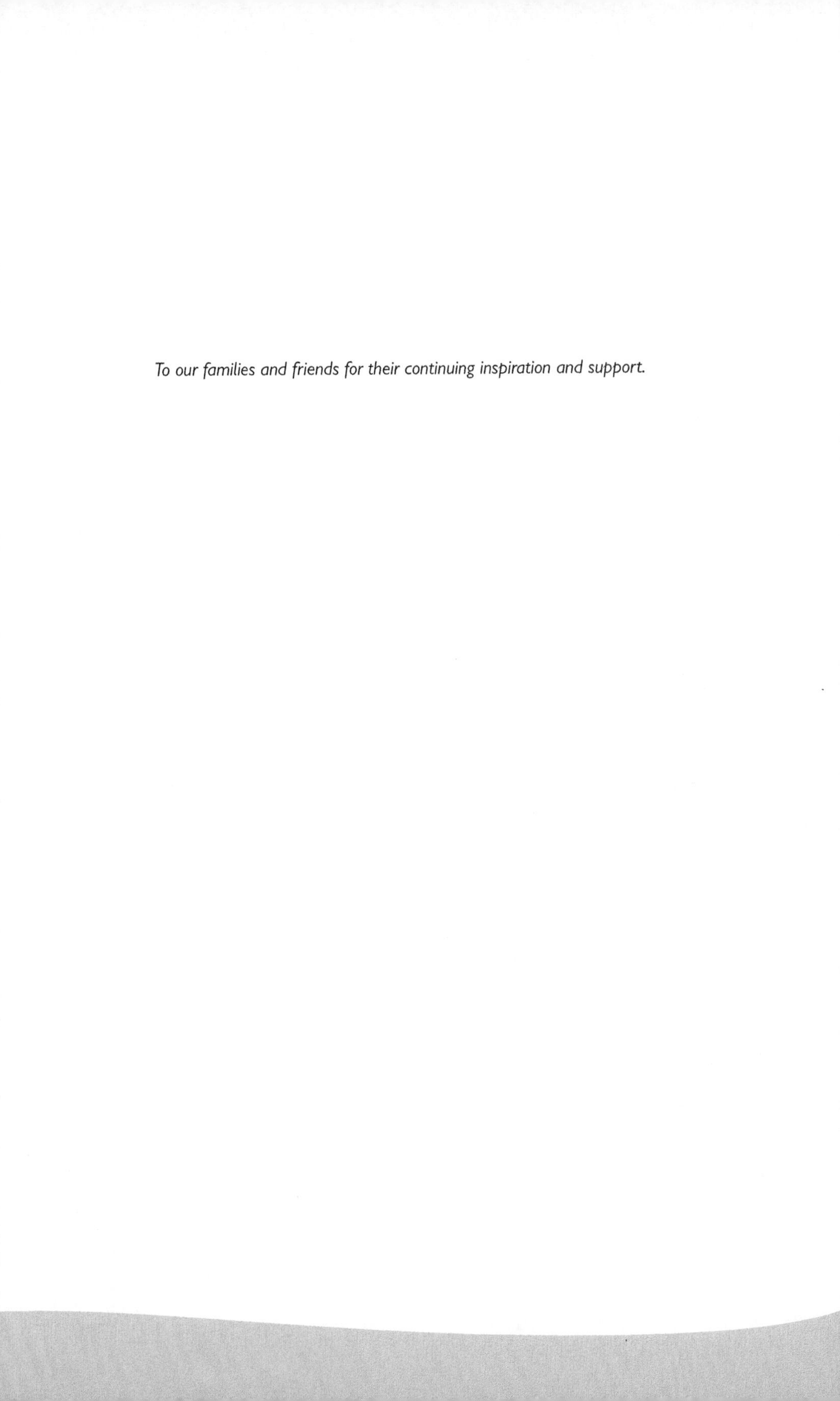

To our families and friends for their continuing inspiration and support.

FOREWORD

The first part of the Fellowship of the Royal College of Radiologists provides a unique challenge to the trainee radiologist. The content that is examined within the physics syllabus is often new and unfamiliar. The introduction of this text is a valuable addition to the existing literature. It covers the established modalities and introduces information and questions about the newest modalities within the radiology field.

Not only is the material comprehensive but the use of additional explanations, diagrams, and learning points provides an excellent reinforcement to the learner.

When used in conjunction with other learning material such as the Royal College of Radiologists e-LD (electronic learning database) it will allow trainees every opportunity to learn and retain the clinically relevant physics material contained within the FRCR First Part curriculum.

Dr Bruce Fox
MBBS MRCP FRCR
PGCertMedEd
Head of Postgraduate School of Radiology
and Consultant GI Radiologist
Derriford Hospital, Plymouth, Devon, UK

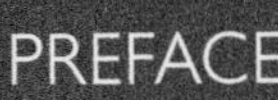

PREFACE

Medical physics is a difficult subject to grasp but remains a crucial first hurdle to aspiring radiologists. During the period of preparation for the first part of the Fellowship of the Royal College of Radiologists (FRCR) Examination, we became aware of the various shortcomings of most recent preparation books, in particular the lack of up-to-date questions. Consequently we have found the need to supplement question books with our own research. As well as this, we felt there was a need to update questions to reflect the recent technological advances such as the advent of Digital Radiography, Multi-detector Computed Tomography, PET as well as recent technical advances in US and MRI—all of which are increasingly being examined by the Royal College. This is reflected by recent changes in the curriculum. We have written this book especially with all these factors in mind.

This book comprehensively covers various topics of medical physics relating to the practice of radiology. It is set out in 11 chapters and contains 400 questions each containing 5 stems. This is a conventional format used by the First FRCR examination. The answer section contains extensive explanations. Trainees from other disciplines such as medical radiography or medical physics may also find this book valuable. It is not a conventional question book in the sense that it also offers a unique revision aid in the way of learning points, tables, and diagrams, which serve to reinforce the learning process. The aims of these small bite-size learning points are to summarize key concepts and facts that as trainees we found most useful during our preparation. This sets it apart from other similar books and we are certain that readers will overwhelmingly benefit from this. Moreover, the answer section is extensively referenced for supplementary reading to the most commonly used textbooks, journal articles, websites, as well as the electronic learning database set up by the Radiology Integrated Training Initiative (R-ITI).

The process of preparing this book has taken a considerable amount of time and effort. We would like to thank all the contributing authors for giving their time, assistance, advice, wisdom, and most importantly their patience in investing in this project. We would also like to thank our Commissioning Editor Chris Reid and Editorial Assistant Stephanie Ireland for their efforts in nurturing this project to fruition. As a result, we are certain that we have come up with the most up-to-date and comprehensive book for the preparation of the First FRCR examination. We hope that it will prove to be a valuable resource for the next generation of radiologists.

V.V
J.J
R.G
R.N
V.S
T.N

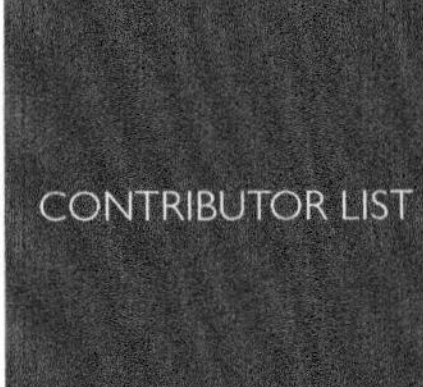

CONTRIBUTOR LIST

Dr Diane De Friend MBChB BSc FRCR
Consultant Radiologist
Derriford Hospital, Plymouth, Devon, UK

Dr Bruce Fox MBBS MRCP FRCR PGCertMedEd
Head of Postgraduate School of Radiology and Consultant GI Radiologist
Derriford Hospital, Plymouth, Devon, UK

Mrs Jacqui George BSc MSc AVS
Vascular Scientist
Vascular Assessment Unit
Derriford Hospital, Plymouth, Devon, UK

Mr Jason Heales BSc MSc MIPEM CSci
Nuclear Medicine Department
Derriford Hospital, Plymouth, Devon, UK

Mr Ivor Jones BSc
Consultant Physicist in Nuclear Medicine
Derriford Hospital, Plymouth, Devon, UK

Mr Robert Loader MSç, BSc DipIPEM(S) CSci
Principal Physicist
Clinical & Radiation Physics Group
Directorate of Healthcare Science & Technology
Derriford Hospital, Plymouth, Devon, UK

Dr Mike Mayo BSc MSc PhD MIPEM MInstP CSci CPhys
Medical Physicist
Head of Clinical Measurements & Innovation
Derriford Hospital, Plymouth, Devon, UK

Mrs Teena Ninan B.Tech M.Tech
Illustrator
Plymouth, Devon, UK

Mr N P Rowles BSc MSc MIPEM MSRP CRadP CSci
Clinical & Radiation Physics
Directorate of Healthcare Science & Technology
Derriford Hospital, Plymouth, Devon, UK

Dr Gregory Stevens DipIPEM(S) MPhys(Hons) MSc PhD
Pre-registration Medical Physicist
Department of Medical Physics and Bioengineering
Derriford Hospital, Plymouth, Devon, UK

CONTENTS

chapter 1

BASIC RADIATION PHYSICS

QUESTIONS

1. Regarding atomic structure:

A. 'Z' is the number of protons in the nucleus.
B. 'A' determines an element's place in the periodic table.
C. A stable nucleus contains equal numbers of protons and neutrons.
D. Neutrons have a relative charge of +1.
E. Protons are loosely bound to neutrons in the nucleus.

2. Concerning orbital electrons:

A. Electrons are arranged in shells around the nucleus at specific energy levels.
B. Binding energy is that required to excite an electron to a higher energy shell.
C. The binding energy is highest for a valence shell electron.
D. Characteristic radiation is produced from the valence shell.
E. K shell binding energy increases with increasing atomic number.

3. Regarding the structure of atoms:

A. A proton has a mass approximately 1850 times that of an electron.
B. An electron is not a nucleon.
C. Positrons have the same mass as electrons.
D. An alpha particle has twice the mass of a proton.
E. There can be up to 8 electrons orbiting the nucleus in the L shell.

4. Nuclides:

A. Are characterized by mass number and atomic number.
B. Are isotopes if they have the same atomic mass but different atomic number.
C. Are radioactive.
D. Have the same chemical properties between isotopes of a particular element.
E. May emit radiation only if they have too many neutrons.

5. Regarding the electromagnetic spectrum:

A. Sound waves fall at the lower end of the spectrum.
B. Velocity of electromagnetic radiation increases as energy increases.
C. Frequency and wavelength of electromagnetic radiation are directly proportional to each other.
D. In a vacuum, velocity of radio waves is equal to that of infrared light.
E. Visible light has a shorter wavelength than ultraviolet light.

6. Electromagnetic radiation:

A. Travels in straight lines if unattenuated.
B. Has wave- and particle-like properties.
C. Has energy that is usually expressed in Joules in diagnostic radiography.
D. Comprises sinusoidally varying electric and magnetic fields perpendicular to each other and to the direction of travel.
E. Includes beta radiation.

7. Ionizing radiation:

A. Causes direct damage if it is absorbed in tissue.
B. Causes indirect damage through ionization of water and production of free radicals.
C. Always obeys the inverse square law.
D. Is useful in medical imaging in all its forms.
E. May require only to be shielded with Perspex.

8. Regarding secondary electrons:

A. They are recoil electrons produced during Compton scattering events.
B. Their range depends only upon the density of the material through which they are travelling.
C. They can interact with inner shell electrons of atoms they pass causing ionization.
D. They are the reason that x-ray and gamma rays are indirectly ionizing.
E. They cause tissue heating.

9. In radioactive decay:

A. Emission of a β^- particle reduces atomic number by 1.
B. Alpha particles are helium nuclei.
C. Some radionuclides emit electrons and characteristic x-rays.
D. Most nuclides left in a metastable state after beta decay, emit gamma rays to reach ground state.
E. Positron emission reduces the number of protons in an atom by 1.

10. Regarding radioactivity:

A. Radioactive decay is the number of disintegrations per minute.
B. Decay rate can be increased by increasing temperature.
C. If stored long enough, the radioactivity of a radionuclide will drop to zero.
D. Beta emission is at a continuous range of energies.
E. Decay constant is the probability of nuclear decay per unit time.

11. The following are true of radionuclides:

A. Physical half-life ($t_{1/2}$) is the time taken for the activity to decay to ½ the original value.
B. Gamma rays are emitted at a single photon energy.
C. Gamma emitting radionuclides with shorter $t_{1/2}$ are safer to use and store than those with longer $t_{1/2}$.
D. In 10 half-lives the activity is reduced by a factor of approximately 1000.
E. Only one type of radiation is emitted by a radionuclide.

12. Direct emission from radioactive decay includes:

A. Beta minus emission.
B. Characteristic x-rays.
C. Bremsstrahlung.
D. Alpha particles.
E. Positron emission.

13. Concerning properties of x-rays:

A. Beam intensity is the total energy per unit area per unit time.
B. The inverse square law applies to all x-ray beams.
C. X-rays have lower linear energy transfer than alpha particles.
D. All electromagnetic radiation can cause ionization.
E. At equivalent energy, an x-ray cannot be distinguished from a gamma ray.

14. Concerning an x-ray tube:

A. Usually a voltage of 10V and a current of 10A pass through the filament.
B. The accelerating voltage of the tube is typically in the range 60–120kV.
C. The process of thermionic emission occurs on the surface of the anode.
D. When an accelerating electron interacts closely with a target nucleus it is deflected and slowed, losing energy that is emitted as an x-ray photon.
E. The angle of the target ensures that all x-rays produced pass through the window in the tube to form a beam.

15. X-ray production in a diagnostic x-ray tube:

A. Occurs when moving electrons interact with target nuclei.
B. Is 99% efficient.
C. Is more efficient with a rotating compared to a stationary anode.
D. Is increased if the target atomic number is increased.
E. Requires a cooling air current at all times within the tube.

16. Radiation output from an x-ray tube increases with:

A. Increasing cathode-to-anode distance.
B. The addition of a filter.
C. Increasing kV.
D. Increasing mA.
E. A constant potential compared to a single phase waveform.

17. In a diagnostic x-ray tube:

A. Heat is only removed to the tube envelope by conduction.
B. The focusing cup is negatively charged.
C. Rotor bearings are lubricated with oil.
D. The anode stem is a poor heat conductor.
E. The addition of rhenium to the tungsten target increases toughness and lifespan of the target.

18. In a diagnostic x-ray tube the anode angle:

A. Is the angle that the target face makes with the x-ray beam.
B. Is the only factor determining focal spot size.
C. Is generally 20–35°.
D. Increases the tube rating if the angle is reduced.
E. Determines the size of field covered by the x-ray beam at a given focus–film distance.

19. The spectrum of an x-ray beam:

A. Is not affected by filtration.
B. Varies with tube current.
C. Has a maximum energy determined by peak tube potential (kVp).
D. Consists of Bremsstrahlung and characteristic radiation if the kVp exceeds the K edge energy of the anode.
E. Has a peak approximately ¾ of the kVp.

20. Regarding an x-ray tube filament:

A. It must have a high melting point and low resistance.
B. Electrons evaporate off through thermionic emission.
C. Tungsten is used because of its high atomic number.
D. It should have a low vapour pressure.
E. It has a negative potential.

21. The anode-heel effect:

A. Produces a uniform x-ray beam across its field.
B. Is more prominent at the cathode end of the tube.
C. Is more noticeable if the focus–film distance is increased.
D. Is greater if the target angle is steeper.
E. Is not used as an advantage in diagnostic radiography.

22. Increasing tube kV (with all other factors constant) increases:

A. Patient entrance surface dose.
B. Scattered compared to primary radiation at the film.
C. Radiographic contrast.
D. Film blackening.
E. Photoelectric interactions compared to Compton interactions.

23. Concerning attenuation of x-rays:

A. Increased tube filtration increases the half value layer.
B. Total attenuation is the product of Compton, photoelectric, and elastic attenuation effects.
C. Half value thickness is inversely proportional to the linear attenuation coefficient.
D. It is altered with differing atomic number materials.
E. It is related to the inverse square law.

24. The half value layer:

A. Is the thickness of a material that will reduce the intensity of a narrow x-ray beam to ¼ of its original value.
B. Is a measure of the penetrating power of an x-ray beam.
C. For lead is greater than for aluminium at a given energy of x-ray beam.
D. Is reduced as the photon energy of the radiation decreases.
E. Will produce exponential attenuation if a narrow x-ray beam passes through successive half value thicknesses of a particular material.

25. The mass attenuation coefficient:

A. Is measured in cm^2/g.
B. Is equal to the linear attenuation coefficient divided by the density.
C. Is less for water than for ice.
D. Has many practical applications in diagnostic radiology.
E. Is proportional to the linear attenuation coefficient.

26. Regarding the linear attenuation coefficient:

A. It is the fractional reduction in intensity per unit thickness.
B. It can be used to calculate the half value thickness.
C. It increases as photon energy increases.
D. It is measured in mm.
E. The greater the difference in linear attenuation coefficients between two tissues, the greater the contrast between them.

27. Regarding scattered radiation:

A. More is measured on the tube side of the patient in diagnostic radiology.
B. A Compton scattered photon is deflected from its path with no loss of energy.
C. There is no ionization with elastic scattering.
D. During a Compton interaction a photoelectron is produced.
E. At higher kV more photons are deflected through large angles.

28. In Compton scattering:

A. There is an interaction with a free electron.
B. The recoil electron can be scattered in any direction.
C. The larger the angle of scatter, the greater the reduction in energy of the incident photon.
D. All the photon's energy can be transferred to the electron.
E. The amount of scatter is proportional to electron density.

29. Concerning the photoelectric effect:

A. The incident photon completely disappears.
B. It is the main attenuation process in bone at 80kV.
C. It may result in scattered radiation.
D. The probability of an interaction increases as photon energy increases.
E. Its contribution to the mass attenuation coefficient increases approximately as the cube of the atomic number.

30. The photoelectric effect:

A. Involves free electrons.
B. Results in the production of characteristic radiation.
C. Only occurs with electrons from the K shell.
D. Is most important at the lower end of the diagnostic range of energies.
E. Results in ionization of the atom.

31. Regarding absorption edges:

A. For a given element, the K-absorption edge is greater than the L-absorption edge.
B. At photon energies just above the K-shell binding energy of an element there is a sharp decrease in the probability of photoelectric interactions.
C. The K-absorption edge is important when choosing an x-ray filter, a contrast medium or an imaging phosphor.
D. An x-ray filter does not transmit photons well if they are of an energy equivalent to its own K-absorption edge.
E. Barium has such a high atomic number that its K-absorption edge does not play a role in diagnostic imaging when it is used as a contrast medium.

32. Filtration of an x-ray beam:

A. Reduces the maximum photon energy (kVp).
B. By the patient is known as inherent filtration.
C. Improves the rating of the x-ray tube.
D. Is more effective for filtering high energy x-rays using a copper rather than an aluminium filter.
E. Results in an image with improved contrast.

33. Inherent filtration of an x-ray tube:

A. Absorbs high energy x-rays.
B. Causes beam hardening.
C. Is usually equivalent to 2.5mm aluminium.
D. Is increased if beryllium instead of glass is used in the tube window.
E. Is mostly due to the oil.

34. Added filtration:

A. Does not affect patient entrance dose.
B. Alters the quality of the x-ray beam.
C. May consist of a compound filter.
D. Is generally made of aluminium in diagnostic tubes.
E. Does not affect the intensity of the beam.

35. X-ray tube rating increases with:

A. Rotating compared to stationary anodes.
B. Larger focal spot size.
C. Increasing the anode angle with fixed focal spot size.
D. Half wave compared to full wave rectification.
E. Quicker production of heat.

36. Measurement of radiation dose:

A. Can be read directly through an electronic read-out from photoconductive silicon diodes.
B. Is useful for personal and patient dosimetry with the use of thermoluminescent dosimeters.
C. May be carried out using thimble ionization chambers within the field of interest.
D. With a dose area product meter provides a figure with the units cGy cm^3.
E. For staff may utilize the photographic effect of silver bromide in a film badge.

37. Regarding ionization chambers:

A. They are used to measure absorbed dose in diagnostic radiography.
B. Ionization of the air in the chamber forms a measurable current by the attraction of the ions to the positive wall of the chamber and negative electrode.
C. Air is convenient for use in the chambers, but is not the ideal material as its effective atomic number is much lower than that of soft tissue.
D. Parallel plate ionization chambers mounted on the collimator of an x-ray tube measure patient dose area product.
E. Any individual ionization chamber may be used accurately over a very wide range of photon energies.

38. Film badges:

A. Use double emulsion film.
B. Are calibrated with a caesium source.
C. Have an open window for the detection of beta particles.
D. Should be analysed once a year when monitoring staff.
E. Use cadmium nuclei to detect neutron exposure.

39. The following are true of thermoluminescent dosimeters:

A. The phosphor used is commonly lithium chloride.
B. X-ray interactions involve outer shell electrons of the thermoluminescent phosphor.
C. When exposed to radiation, interactions excite electrons that become trapped in the forbidden energy band.
D. The amount of light produced depends on the energy of the photons involved in the exposure.
E. Their response is linear with dose over a wide range.

40. Regarding luminescence:

A. It is the process by which a material absorbs energy from an external source and re-emits it as light.
B. Fluorescence is the delayed emission of light following energy input.
C. For light to be emitted from a phosphor, electrons in the electron traps must fall to the conduction band.
D. After irradiation, a thermoluminescent phosphor must be stimulated with a laser for light to be emitted.
E. Intensity of light emitted from a phosphor is proportional to the intensity of the irradiating x-ray beam.

chapter 1

BASIC RADIATION PHYSICS

ANSWERS

1. A. True: Z is the atomic number and indicates the number of protons in the nucleus.
B. False: A is the mass number. Z determines place in the periodic table.
C. False: Higher atomic number nuclei require more neutrons than protons for stability.
D. False: Neutrons have no charge, protons +1.
E. False: They are tightly bound.

Allisy-Roberts & Williams. *Farr's Physics for Medical Imaging*, 2nd edn, Saunders Elsevier, 2008. pp. 1–3.

2. A. True.
B. False: Binding energy is expended completely removing the electron from the atom.
C. False: It is lowest for valence shell electrons and highest for the K shell.
D. False: Characteristic radiation is from inner shells. The valence shell gives the chemical properties.
E. True.

Allisy-Roberts & Williams. *Farr's Physics for Medical Imaging*, 2nd edn, Saunders Elsevier, 2008. pp. 1–3.

3. A. True.
B. True: Neutrons and protons are nucleons.
C. True.
D. False: Alpha particles consist of 2 protons and 2 neutrons (helium nucleus), therefore the mass is 4 times that of a proton.
E. True: There can be up to 2 electrons in the K shell, 8 in the L shell, 18 in the M shell and 32 in the N shell.

Allisy-Roberts & Williams. *Farr's Physics for Medical Imaging*, 2nd edn, Saunders Elsevier, 2008. pp. 1–3.
Electronic Learning Database, E-Learning for Healthcare, Radiology—Integrated Training Initiative (R-ITI).www.e-lfh.org.uk
Module: 8a_001: Atomic Structure.

Table 1.1 shows information regarding constituents of the atom.

Table 1.1 Constituents of an atom

	Relative Charge	Relative Mass
Neutron	0	1
Proton	+1	1
Electron	−1	0.00054
Positron	+1	0.00054
Alpha Particle	+2	4

4. A. True: Each particular combination of Z and A defines a nuclide.
B. False: Nuclides with the same number of protons but different number of neutrons are isotopes, therefore they have the same atomic number and different atomic mass.
C. False: Not all are radioactive.
D. True: Isotopes have the same number of protons and therefore when neutral the same number of electrons.
E. False: Too few or too many.

Allisy-Roberts & Williams. *Farr's Physics for Medical Imaging*, 2nd edn, Saunders Elsevier, 2008. pp. 121–2.
Electronic Learning Database, E-Learning for Healthcare, Radiology—Integrated Training Initiative (R-ITI).www.e-lfh.org.uk
Module: 8a_002: Radioactivity.

5. A. False: Sound waves do not fall within the spectrum.
B. False: Frequency increases with energy, but velocity is constant.
C. True.
D. True: All electromagnetic radiation travels at the speed of light in a vacuum.
E. False: UV light is further up the spectrum, therefore has a shorter wavelength than visible light.

Electronic Learning Database, E-Learning for Healthcare, Radiology—Integrated Training Initiative (R-ITI).www.e-lfh.org.uk
Module: 8a_006: Electromagnetic Radiation.

6. A. True.
B. True.
C. False: Electron volts (eV), which give manageable numbers for calculations ($1\text{eV} = 1.6 \times 10^{-19}$ Joules).
D. True.
E. False: Beta particles are electrons emitted from the nucleus.

Electronic Learning Database, E-Learning for Healthcare, Radiology—Integrated Training Initiative (R-ITI).www.e-lfh.org.uk
Module: 8a_020: Biological Effects Interaction of Radiation with Tissue.

Learning Points

Table 1.2 Distinction between atomic and mass numbers

Z	Atomic number
	Number of protons
	Number of electrons
A	Mass number
	Number of protons + netrons

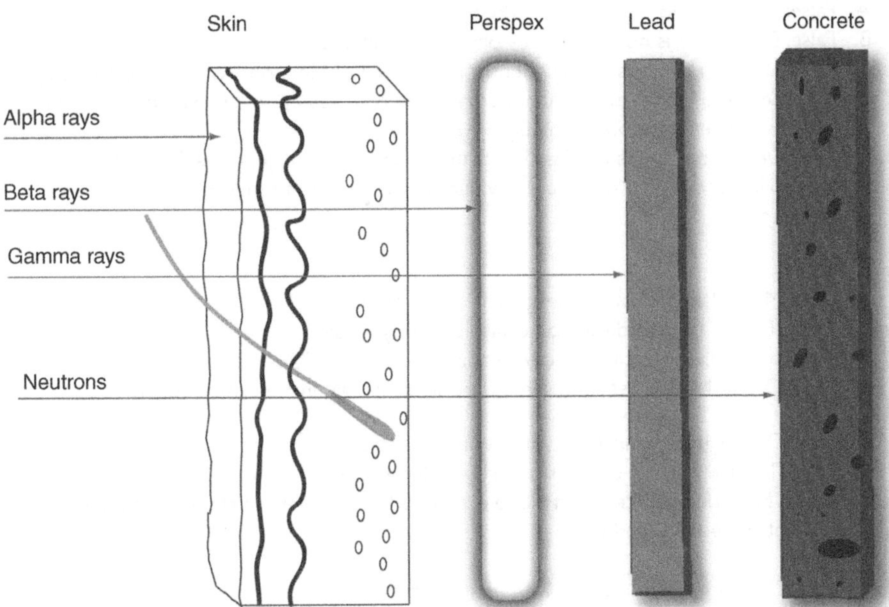

Figure 1.1 Attenuation properties of different types of radiation

7. A. True.
B. True.
C. False: Only applicable to types of electromagnetic radiation from a point source and without attenuation.
D. False: Gamma and x-rays are useful, neutrons, alpha, and beta particles are not.
E. True: Beta radiation may require only Perspex shielding, however optimal shielding is achieved with Perspex backed with lead.

8. A. True.
B. False: Range also depends upon their initial energy.
C. False: They interact with outer shell electrons to cause ionization.
D. True: Alpha and beta particles are directly ionizing as they are charged.
E. True: Energy from the x-ray beam is converted into increased molecular motion and therefore heat.

Allisy-Roberts & Williams. *Farr's Physics for Medical Imaging*, 2nd edn, Saunders Elsevier, 2008. pp. 11–14.

9. A. False: A neutron converts to a proton and a β^- particle, therefore atomic number increases by 1.
B. True.
C. True: During internal conversion a K shell electron is ejected, producing characteristic x-rays when the K shell vacancy is filled with an electron from the L shell.
D. True: This is isomeric transition.
E. True: A proton converts to a neutron and a β^+ particle, therefore atomic number decreases by 1.

Further Reading. Allisy-Roberts & Williams. *Farr's Physics for Medical Imaging*, 2nd edn, Saunders Elsevier, 2008. pp. 121–2.

10. A. False: Disintegrations per second (Bequerels (Bq)).
B. False: Decay rate is not affected by physical conditions.
C. True: Although decay is an exponential process, all of the atoms will eventually decay.
D. True: Beta emission is at a continuous range of energies up to a maximum (E_{max}), and with average energy approximately $E_{max}/3$.
E. True: Decay constant is the fraction of nuclei decaying per unit time. This is the probability of decay, as decay of individual atoms occurs at random and cannot be predicted.

11. A. True.
B. False: More than 1 photon energy may be emitted.
C. True: Shorter time to decay to negligible activity is safer.
D. True: 10 half lives indicates decay by a factor of 2^{10} or 1024.
E. False: Often there is beta and gamma, or alpha and gamma emission together.

12. A. True: Occurs in radionuclides with neutron excess.
B. True: Through internal conversion or K-shell capture.
C. False: This is due to interactions of electrons with the electric field around the nucleus and not of decay directly.
D. True.
E. True: Occurs in radionuclides with neutron deficit.

13. A. True: This is the energy fluence rate or intensity.
B. False: This only applies to x-rays from a point source.
C. True: Alpha particles are heavy and produce ionizing events closely spaced along a short path, causing maximum DNA damage.
D. False: Only high-energy photons (x-rays/gamma rays) are ionizing.
E. True: How they are produced differs, but they are indistinguishable at equivalent energies.

Electronic Learning Database, E-Learning for Healthcare, Radiology—Integrated Training Initiative (R-ITI).www.e-lfh.org.uk
Module: 8a_0003: Basics of X-ray Production.
Module: 8a_004: Interaction of X and Gamma Rays with Matter.

14. A. True: This heats the filament to incandescence, so that electrons can be boiled off by thermionic emission in order to be accelerated across the tube.
B. True: This is the tube potential that drives the electron stream from cathode to anode.
C. False: It occurs at the surface of the cathode.
D. True: This is Bremsstrahlung, or braking radiation, which results in the continuous spectrum of radiation.
E. False: X-rays will be produced in many directions, but only those that pass through the window will contribute to the useful beam, the others will be absorbed by the tube housing.

Sherer, Visconti, Ritenour. *Radiation Protection in Medical Radiography*, 4th edn, Mosby, 2002. pp. 25–6.

15. A. True: Continuous spectrum radiation (Bremsstrahlung) is produced through electron–nucleus interactions, and characteristic radiation is produced through electron–electron interactions within the target.
B. False: Approximately 99% heat production, 1% x-ray production.
C. True.
D. True: Higher atomic number nuclei have increased electric field, therefore there are more x-ray-producing interactions.
E. False: The tube contains a vacuum.

Allisy-Roberts & Williams. *Farr's Physics for Medical Imaging*, 2nd edn, Saunders Elsevier, 2008. pp. 5–6.

16. A. False: No relation.
B. False: Decreases total output.
C. True: Output is approximately proportional to kV^2.
D. True: Output is proportional to mA.
E. True: kV is near its maximum for longer.

17. A. False: Heat is radiated through the vacuum to the envelope.
B. True: To repel electrons from the filament and produce a narrow beam.
C. False: Silver is used—oil would evaporate in the vacuum.
D. True: Prevents damage to the rotor assembly.
E. True: This alloy reduces surface pitting and increases lifespan.

18. A. True.
B. False: The size of the filament also determines focal spot size.
C. False: The angle is generally 7–20°.
D. True.
E. True: The steeper the angle, the narrower the x-ray beam and the smaller field covered.

19. A. False: Filtration removes low energy photons, hardening the beam and increasing the mean energy of the spectrum.
B. False: Increasing mA merely increases the number of photons. Their energy and therefore the shape of the spectrum remains the same if kV is unaltered.
C. True: Peak potential gives the electrons striking the target their peak energy, therefore dictating peak photon energy in the x-ray beam.
D. True: Bremsstrahlung is the continuous spectrum, and characteristic radiation the peaks specific to the anode material.
E. False: The spectrum peak is ⅓ to ½kVp, whereas average or effective energy is 50–60% of the maximum.

Allisy-Roberts & Williams. *Farr's Physics for Medical Imaging*, 2nd edn, Saunders Elsevier, 2008. pp. 9–16.

20. A. False: High melting point and high resistance to generate heat for thermionic emission.
B. True: Filament heat allows electrons to boil off and create space charge around the cathode that can be accelerated towards the anode.
C. False: This is the reason that it is chosen for the anode.
D. True: A good property for thermionic emission.
E. True: The focusing cup is usually more negative than the filament.

21. A. False: Photons on the anode side of the beam have more target material to travel through, so are attenuated and the intensity reduced.
B. False: By definition it is the 'anode' heel effect.
C. False: With increased distance the beam diverges further and the film only intercepts the central part of the beam.
D. True: The steeper the target, the further through the target material the photons on the anode side of the beam have to travel and the more attenuated they are.
E. False: It is used in mammography and extremity radiography, where a thicker part of the body is placed towards the cathode side.

Allisy-Roberts & Williams. *Farr's Physics for Medical Imaging*, 2nd edn, Saunders Elsevier, 2008. pp. 58 and 62.

22. A. True.
B. True: Higher kV x-rays are more penetrating so scattering events occur deeper in the patient nearer the film. Also, the scattered photons are more penetrating.
C. False: Contrast decreases as kV increases.
D. True: Increased kV causes increased exposure and increased film density.
E. False: At higher kVs Compton events are favoured.

23. A. True: Through beam hardening.
B. True: This is the total attenuation. Attenuation coefficient is the sum of each process.
C. True: Half value layer is 0.69/μ (μ = linear attenuation coefficient = fraction of the primary beam that is removed per unit distance).
D. True: Attenuation is increased with increasing Z number and increasing density of the attenuating material, through increased Compton scatter and photoelectric absorption. (The probability of photoelectric absorption $\propto Z^3$).
E. False: Attenuation is the reduction in intensity due to interactions in matter, whereas the inverse square law is the reduction in intensity due to beam divergence from a point source.

Allisy-Roberts & Williams. *Farr's Physics for Medical Imaging*, 2nd edn, Saunders Elsevier, 2008. pp. 9–11.

24. A. False: It is the thickness of a material that reduces intensity to half its original value.
B. True.
C. False: The HVL decreases as the atomic number of the attenuating material increases.
D. True.
E. True.

Allisy-Roberts & Williams. *Farr's Physics for Medical Imaging*, 2nd edn, Saunders Elsevier, 2008. pp. 9–11.

25. A. True.
B. True.
C. False: It is equal for water and ice, as it is independent of physical density.
D. False: The linear attenuation coefficient has more practical applications, as film density produced by a certain depth of tissue is more useful than that produced by a certain mass of tissue.
E. True.

Allisy-Roberts & Williams. *Farr's Physics for Medical Imaging*, 2nd edn, Saunders Elsevier, 2008. pp. 9–11.

26. A. True.
B. True: HVT equals 0.693 divided by the linear attenuation coefficient.
C. False: It decreases as photon energy increases.
D. False: mm^{-1}.
E. True: Contrast is proportional to the product of the difference between the 2 linear attenuation coefficients and the thickness of the tissues involved.

Allisy-Roberts & Williams. *Farr's Physics for Medical Imaging*, 2nd edn, Saunders Elsevier, 2008. pp. 9–11.

27. A. True: Most interactions occur at the entrance surface of the patient and forward scattered photons are more attenuated than backscattered ones.
B. False: This is elastic scattering.
C. True.
D. False: These are formed in photoelectric interactions.
E. False: Within the diagnostic range there is slight increase in forward scatter as kV increases, therefore there are more small angle deflections.

Sherer, Visconti, Ritenour. *Radiation Protection in Medical Radiography*, 4th edn, Mosby, 2002. pp. 30–9.
Allisy-Roberts & Williams. *Farr's Physics for Medical Imaging*, 2nd edn, Saunders Elsevier, 2008. pp. 11–15.

28. A. True: The incident photon interacts with an outer shell an electron.
B. False: The scattered photon can be emitted in any direction, but the recoil electron can be projected only forwards or sideways.
C. True.
D. False: The photon is scattered and therefore still retains some energy. Total absorption occurs in photoelectric interactions.
E. True: The greater the concentration of electrons, the greater the probability of an interaction.

Sherer, Visconti, Ritenour. *Radiation Protection in Medical Radiography*, 4th edn, Mosby, 2002. pp. 30–9.

29. A. True.
B. False: The photoelectric effect predominates over Compton scatter in bone below 50kV and in soft tissue below 30kV.
C. False: The photon is always completely absorbed.
D. False: The probability of photoelectric interaction is inversely proportional to photon energy cubed.
E. True: The probability of photoelectric interaction $\propto Z^3$.

Sherer, Visconti, Ritenour. *Radiation Protection in Medical Radiography*, 4th edn, Mosby, 2002. pp. 30–9.

30. A. False: It involves inner shell electrons.
B. True: The ejection of a photoelectron by the incident photon allows an outer shell electron to fall into the gap, with the emission of photons of characteristic radiation.
C. False: Can also occur with the L shell.
D. True.
E. True: As an electron is removed a net negative charge results.

Sherer, Visconti, Ritenour. *Radiation Protection in Medical Radiography*, 4th edn, Mosby, 2002. pp. 30–9.

31. A. True: K-shell binding energy is always greater than the L-shell binding energy for a given element.
B. False: There is a sharp increase in the probability of photoelectric interactions just above the K-shell binding energy.
C. True.
D. False: It will be relatively transparent to photons of the energy of its absorption edge.
E. False: The atomic number of barium is 56 and the K-absorption edge is 37keV. Diagnostic x-ray beams contain a high proportion of photons around this energy, ensuring a high probability of photoelectric interactions.

Allisy-Roberts & Williams. *Farr's Physics for Medical Imaging*, 2nd edn, Saunders Elsevier, 2008. p. 58.

32. A. False: The kVp remains the same, but lower energy photons are filtered out and average kV increases.
B. False: Inherent filtration results from absorption of x-rays as they pass through the tube.
C. False: Tube loading is increased due to the reduced intensity of the x-ray beam once it has passed through the filter.
D. True: Copper has a higher atomic number than aluminium, so is better at filtering higher energy x-rays.
E. False: Filtration hardens the beam by increasing the mean energy of the photons, therefore contrast in the image is decreased.

Sherer, Visconti, Ritenour. *Radiation Protection in Medical Radiography*, 4th edn, Mosby, 2002. pp. 163–6.
Allisy-Roberts & Williams. *Farr's Physics for Medical Imaging*, 2nd edn, Saunders Elsevier, 2008. pp. 15–16.

33. A. False: Absorbs low energy x-rays.
B. True: By removing low energy photons and increasing the average energy of the beam.
C. False: Total filtration is approximately 2.5mm Al, inherent is 0.5–1mm.
D. False: Beryllium has a lower atomic number than glass, therefore filtration is less.
E. False: Due to target, tube window, and the oil.

Sherer, Visconti, Ritenour. *Radiation Protection in Medical Radiography*, 4th edn, Mosby, 2002. pp. 163–6.

34. A. False: Low energy photons are removed, which would contribute to patient dose, but not to the image.
B. True: As mean kV is increased, penetrating power and therefore quality increases.
C. True: Copper is used with a backing of aluminium on the patient side to absorb the 9kV characteristic radiation from the copper.
D. True.
E. False: Intensity or amount of radiation is decreased by the filter.

Allisy-Roberts & Williams. *Farr's Physics for Medical Imaging*, 2nd edn, Saunders Elsevier, 2008. pp. 15–16.

35. A. True: There is more efficient heat loss from a rotating anode, so the rating is higher.
B. True: A larger focal spot causes less heating than if the beam were focused onto a smaller area.
C. False: A smaller anode angle has a higher heat rating.
D. False: Rating is increased with full wave rectification.
E. False: This makes the tube rating lower.

Allisy-Roberts & Williams. *Farr's Physics for Medical Imaging*, 2nd edn, Saunders Elsevier, 2008. pp. 60–1.
Electronic Learning Database, E-Learning for Healthcare, Radiology—Integrated Training Initiative (R-ITI).www.e-lfh.org.uk
Module: 8a_063: Heat Removal (Thermal Loading).

36. A. True: Useful for personal dosimeters and quality assurance.
B. True.
C. True.
D. False: It is the product of dose and area with units cGy cm^2.
E. True.

Sherer, Visconti, Ritenour. *Radiation Protection in Medical Radiography*, 4th edn, Mosby, 2002. pp. 225–42.

37. A. True: They measure air kerma (kinetic energy released to matter), which at diagnostic energies is effectively equal to absorbed dose.
B. True.
C. False: It is ideal, as the effective atomic number of air is 7.6, and that of soft tissue is 7.4.
D. True.
E. False: Lower energy beams (such as in mammography) require ionization chambers with thinner walls to avoid undue attenuation of radiation by the chamber.

38. A. True: If the fast emulsion is over-exposed by a high-dose exposure, the slow emulsion can be read.
B. True.
C. True.
D. False: They are subject to environmental effects, so should not be used for longer than a month.
E. True: The interaction of neutrons with the cadmium nuclei results in gamma ray emission that is detected by the film.

Sherer, Visconti, Ritenour. *Radiation Protection in Medical Radiography*, 4th edn, Mosby, 2002. pp. 225–42.
Electronic Learning Database, E-Learning for Healthcare, Radiology—Integrated Training Initiative (R-ITI).www.e-lfh.org.uk
Module: 8a_052: Personal Dosimetry.

39. A. False: Lithium fluoride.
B. True: Valence shell electrons are involved.
C. True: A valence shell electron is excited into the conduction band and then falls back into an electron trap in the forbidden energy band.
D. True.
E. True.

Sherer, Visconti, Ritenour. *Radiation Protection in Medical Radiography*, 4th edn, Mosby, 2002. pp. 225–42.
Electronic Learning Database, E-Learning for Healthcare, Radiology—Integrated Training Initiative (R-ITI).www.e-lfh.org.uk
Module: 8a_052: Personal Dosimetry.

40. A. True.
B. False: Fluorescence is the instantaneous emission of light following energy input, phosphorescence is the delayed emission of light.
C. False: The x-ray photons excite electrons from the valence band to the conduction band, where they then fall into electron traps. They must fall back to the valence band for light to be emitted.
D. False: Thermoluminescence requires heating, photostimulable luminescence requires light.
E. True.

Allisy-Roberts & Williams. *Farr's Physics for Medical Imaging*, 2nd edn, Saunders Elsevier, 2008. pp. 19–20.

chapter 2

GENERAL RADIATION HAZARDS AND PROTECTION

QUESTIONS

1. Deterministic effects of ionizing radiation include:

A. Cataract
B. Epilation
C. Leukaemia
D. Lung cancer
E. Erythema

2. Stochastic effects of radiation include:

A. Infertility
B. Leukaemia
C. Cataract
D. Cancer
E. Hair loss

3. Equivalent dose:

A. Is derived from absorbed dose multiplied by a tissue weighting factor.
B. Is measured in Sieverts (Sv).
C. Is averaged over all tissues of the body.
D. Is the same as absorbed dose for neutrons.
E. Takes into account sensitivity of the tissues to radiation.

4. Absorbed dose

A. Relative to an organ depends on its mass.
B. Is measured in Joules/Kg.
C. Is measured in Sieverts.
D. Depends on the radiation weighting factor.
E. Is the amount of energy deposited per unit mass to a medium.

5. Effective dose

A. Is derived from absorbed dose multiplied by a tissue weighting factor.
B. Is measured in Gray.
C. Takes into consideration the different radiosensitivity of tissues.
D. Combines organ doses to give a whole body dose.
E. In a dental film is in the order of 0.004mSv.

6. Regarding ionizing radiation

A. Neutrons are low LET (linear energy transfer) radiation.
B. The radiation weighting factor for alpha particles is 20.
C. X-rays and beta particles have the same radiation weighting factor.
D. The radiation weighting factor for neutrons is unity.
E. For x-rays absorbed dose is equal to the equivalent dose.

7. The following tissues have a *high* carcinogenic risk from radiation (more than or equal to 0.12 tissue-specific weighting factor):

A. Colon
B. Skin
C. Breast
D. Bone marrow
E. Oesophagus

8. The following tissues have a *moderate* carcinogenic risk from radiation (0.05 in tissue-specific weighting factor):

A. Skin
B. Gonads
C. Lung
D. Breast
E. Bone

9. The tissue-specific weighting factors are true for the following organs:

A. Bone—0.05
B. Breast—0.12
C. Gonads—0.12
D. Thyroid—0.05
E. Skin—0.01

10. The units for the following terms are true:

A. Entrance surface dose (ESD)—Sv
B. Equivalent dose—Gy
C. Dose area product (DAP)—Gy cm
D. Absorbed dose—Joules/kg
E. Effective dose—Gy

11. Regarding deterministic effects:

A. Diarrhoea and vomiting are examples.
B. There is a threshold dose above which they do not occur.
C. Effects occur by chance.
D. The threshold dose is the same for different deterministic effects.
E. Severity increases with increasing dose.

12. Regarding stochastic effects:

A. The probability of a stochastic effect is independent of dose.
B. Occur immediately after exposure to ionising radiation.
C. Have a linear no threshold theory.
D. Sterility is an example.
E. Breast cancer is an example.

13. Regarding deterministic and stochastic effects of radiation:

A. In the daily practice of diagnostic radiology stochastic effects are commoner than deterministic effects.
B. The chances of producing deterministic effects is the same for x-rays and gamma rays.
C. No dose is considered safe for deterministic effects.
D. Deterministic effects may be non-additive.
E. Skin necrosis is an example of a stochastic effect.

14. Regarding ionizing radiation:

A. Beta particles travel through matter at high speeds.
B. Alpha particles travel through matter at low speeds.
C. Alpha particles are similar to the nucleus of hydrogen.
D. Beta particles are heavier than alpha particles.
E. Alpha particles have useful applications in diagnostic radiology.

15. The following entrance surface doses are typical for the following examinations:

A. PA chest film—0.15mGy.
B. Lateral lumbar spine x-ray—12mGy.
C. AP skull x-ray—2mGy.
D. AP abdomen film—8mGy.
E. Fluoroscopy dose rate—100–150mGy/min.

16. The effective doses are typical for the following examinations:

A. CT head—2mSv
B. PA chest film—0.15mSv
C. CT chest—4mSv
D. Barium enema—7mSv
E. Lumbar spine x-rays—0.8mSv

17. Regarding radiation interactions with tissue:

A. Biological damage to tissue occurs immediately on interaction with tissue.
B. Molecular damage to tissue occurs hours after interaction with tissues.
C. Chemical changes in tissue occurs hours after interaction.
D. The principal radiation sources for medical exposures is x-rays and gamma radiation.
E. Depends on the radiosensitivity of tissues.

18. Regarding biological effects of ionizing radiation:

A. Direct damage to tissue occurs by the production of free radicals.
B. Indirect damage to tissue occurs by the rupture of covalent bonds.
C. Cell death occurs when there is insufficient time for tissues to recover between subsequent irradiation events.
D. Free radicals produced secondary to ionization causes chemical changes in tissues.
E. Is independent of the type of ionizing radiation.

19. The threshold doses for the following deterministic effects are typical:

A. Cataract—5Gy
B. Hair loss—2–5Gy
C. Transient erythema—2Gy
D. Sterility—2–6Gy
E. Depression of haematopoiesis— >0.5Gy

20. The potential risks to the foetus from radiation in utero include:

A. Development of cancer
B. Mental retardation
C. Decrease in IQ
D. Intrauterine growth retardation
E. Leukaemia

21. The potential for the following foetal risks is maximum if radiation received in utero is at the following times:

A. Foetal abnormalities—3rd to 8th week of pregnancy.
B. Mental retardation—8th to 15th week of pregnancy.
C. Foetal death—1st trimester.
D. Childhood cancers—3rd trimester.
E. Growth retardation—8th to 25th week of pregnancy.

22. Regarding the effects of ionizing radiation:

A. The risk of fatal cancer from a uniform whole body irradiation is 1 in 200,000 per mSv.
B. The risk of developing fatal childhood cancer from irradiation in utero is 1 in 50,000 per mGy.
C. The cornea is more radiosensitive than the lens.
D. Radiation dose to the hands of staff arises from the use of radionuclides as well as from x-rays.
E. Deterministic effects are hereditary.

23. Regarding the natural and artificial sources of radiation:

A. Sodium is the commonest contributor of radiation from internal sources.
B. The average dose of radiation to the UK population from natural sources is 1.7mSv per year.
C. The average dose of radiation to the population in Cornwall from natural sources is 3 times that of the average for the rest of the UK.
D. The decay of radon is primarily associated with the emission of gamma rays.
E. The dose received from medical diagnostic procedures averaged over the whole population in the UK is 250μSv.

24. Dose area product (DAP):

A. Can be measured with a thermo luminescent dosimeter (TLD).
B. Decreases with the square of the distance from the x-ray focus.
C. Is an appropriate quantity for dosimetry in fluoroscopy.
D. Is an appropriate quantity for dosimetry in CT.
E. May be used to set diagnostic reference levels.

25. Entrance surface dose (ESD):

A. Is measured in Gycm^2.
B. Increases in proportion to x-ray field size.
C. Can be calculated from knowledge of exposure factors and x-ray output data.
D. Can be measured from DAP if the x-ray field size and back scatter are known.
E. Can be measured using a TLD.

26. Regarding thermoluminescent dosimeters:

A. They are generally used in conjunction with filters.
B. They contain a crystal of lithium iodide.
C. They have a linear response over a wide dose range.
D. They can differentiate between radiation types.
E. They can measure dose rate.

27. Advantages of thermoluminescent dosimeters:

A. They can be reused.
B. The sensitivity is significantly better than film.
C. They can be used to measure both shallow and deep doses.
D. They can measure dose rates.
E. They can be used to monitor eye doses.

28. Film badges:

A. Are able to identify the type of exposure.
B. Utilize a single sided film emulsion.
C. Are relatively resistant to environmental effects.
D. Utilize a double sided film emulsion with screen.
E. Have a sensitivity similar to TLDs.

29. Regarding personal dosimeters:

A. TLDs can provide a direct reading of dose.
B. TLDs provide a permanent record of dose.
C. Film badges do not require calibration.
D. Aluminium oxide is used in optical stimulated luminescent dosimeters.
E. Optical stimulated luminescent dosimeters give readings down to 0.01mSv.

30. Thermoluminescent dosimeters

A. Are used for assessment of finger doses.
B. Are relatively cheaper than film badges.
C. Are used to detect radioactive contamination.
D. The dose can be read only once.
E. Are unaffected by environmental effects.

31. Thermoluminescent dosimeters:

A. An immediate read out is possible.
B. Sensitivity is relatively energy dependent.
C. TLD crystal needs to be heated to about 300°C to be read.
D. TLDs need to be annealed after read out.
E. TLD crystal can be calcium fluoride.

32. Film badges:

A. Sensitivity is about 0.1–0.2mSv.
B. Can be used for assessment of finger dose.
C. Provide a permanent record of exposure.
D. Are usually replaced 3 monthly.
E. Measure the effective dose received.

33. Regarding personal dosimeters:

A. TLDs have a precision better than 1%.
B. TLDs can be used to measure dose to a patient.
C. Dose to a patient can be measured with an ionization chamber.
D. Geiger Muller counters require a quenching agent.
E. The outer case of the Geiger Muller counter is the anode.

34. Electronic personal dosimeters:

A. Are more than 100 times sensitive than TLDs.
B. Measure both dose and dose rates.
C. Have sensitivity to the nearest 1μSv.
D. Do not provide a direct reading.
E. The silicone diode detector is a common type.

35. Regarding personal dosimeters:

A. TLD should not be used without a dosimeter holder.
B. During interventional procedures the TLD must be worn above the protective lead apron.
C. Electronic personal dosimeters are used to detect radioactive contamination.
D. The TLD holder helps to differentiate between skin doses and deeper doses.
E. The precision of a TLD is approximately 15% for low doses.

36. Geiger Muller tubes:

A. Have a dead time when no reading can be done.
B. Are used mainly for patient monitoring.
C. Detect all types of radiation.
D. Can distinguish between all types of radiation.
E. Contain a central wire cathode.

chapter 2

GENERAL RADIATION HAZARDS AND PROTECTION

ANSWERS

1. A. True.
B. True.
C. False.
D. False.
E. True.

Allisy-Roberts & Williams. *Farr's Physics for Medical Imaging*, 2nd edn, Saunders Elsevier, 2008. pp. 25–6.
Sherer, Visconti, and Ritenour. *Radiation Protection in Medical Radiography*, 4th edn, Mosby, 2002. pp. 73–4.

2. A. False.
B. True.
C. False.
D. True.
E. False.

Allisy-Roberts & Williams. *Farr's Physics for Medical Imaging*, 2nd edn, Saunders Elsevier, 2008. pp. 26–7.
Sherer, Visconti, and Ritenour. *Radiation Protection in Medical Radiography*, 4th edn, Mosby, 2002. pp. 73–4.
Table 2.1 summarizes the differences between deterministic and stochastic effects.

Table 2.1 The differences between deterministic and stochasitc effects

Deterministic	Stochastic
Damage depends on absorbed dose	Severity is independent of absorbed dose
Threshold exists	Threshold does not exist
	Probability of occurrence depends on absorbed dose
Examples: cataract, erythema, infertility	Examples: radiation-induced cancer, genetic effect

3. A. False: It is derived from absorbed dose multiplied by a radiation weighting factor.
B. True.
C. False.
D. False: As the radiation weighting factor for neutrons range from 5 to 20.
E. False: Effective dose takes into account the sensitivity of tissues to radiation.

Allisy-Roberts & Williams. *Farr's Physics for Medical Imaging*, 2nd edn, Saunders Elsevier, 2008. pp. 24–5.
Sherer, Visconti, and Ritenour. *Radiation Protection in Medical Radiography*, 4th edn, Mosby, 2002. pp. 51–2.

4. A. False.
B. True: The unit is Gray & 1 Gray = 1 Joule/Kg.
C. False.
D. False.
E. True.

Allisy-Roberts & Williams. *Farr's Physics for Medical Imaging*, 2nd edn, Saunders Elsevier, 2008. pp. 16–17.
Sherer, Visconti, and Ritenour. *Radiation Protection in Medical Radiography*, 4th edn, Mosby, 2002. pp. 51–62.

5. A. False: It is derived from equivalent dose multiplied by a tissue weighting factor.
B. False: It is measured in Sieverts.
C. True.
D. True.
E. True.

Allisy-Roberts & Williams. *Farr's Physics for Medical Imaging*, 2nd edn, Saunders Elsevier, 2008. pp. 25–28.
Sherer, Visconti, and Ritenour. *Radiation Protection in Medical Radiography*, 4th edn, Mosby, 2002. pp. 51–62.
See Table 2.2 for different types of doses.

6. A. False: Neutrons are high-LET radiation.
B. True.
C. True: The radiation weighting factor for both is unity.
D. False: It is 5–20 depending on the radiation energy.
E. True: Equivalent dose = Absorbed dose × Radiation weighting factor and the radiation weighting factor for x-rays is 1.

Sherer, Visconti, and Ritenour. *Radiation Protection in Medical Radiography*, 4th edn, Mosby, 2002. pp. 51–62.
Table 2.3 summarizes radiation weighting factors

Learning Points

Table 2.2 Different types of doses

	Definition	Units
Absorbed Dose	Energy deposited per unit mass	Joules/Kg(J/kg) Gray (Gy)
Equivalent Dose	Absorbed dose x radiation weighting factor	Sieverts (Sv)
Effective Dose	Equivalent dose x tissue weighting factor for all tissues	Milisieverts (mSV)

Table 2.3 Radiation weighting factors

Radiation	Radiation weighting factor
X-rays	1
Gamma rays	1
Beta particles	1
Positrons	1
Neutrons	5–20
Alpha particles	20

Table 2.4 Organ-/tissue-specific weighting factors (W_T)

Organ/Tissue	Weighting factor (W_T)	
Gonads	0.2	High
Stomach	0.12	High
Colon	0.12	High
Lung	0.12	High
Red bone marrow	0.12	High
Breast	0.12	High
Oesophagus	0.05	Medium
Bladder	0.05	Medium
Liver	0.05	Medium
Thyroid	0.05	Medium
Bone	0.01	Low
Skin	0.01	Low
Remainder	0.05	Low

Adapted from ICRP-103.

7. A. True.
B. False.
C. True: According to ICRP-103 (2005), breast is classified as high carcinogenic risk from radiation with a tissue-specific weighting factor of 0.12.
D. True.
E. False.

Allisy-Roberts & Williams. *Farr's Physics for Medical Imaging*, 2nd edn, Saunders Elsevier, 2008. pp. 27–28.
Sherer, Visconti, and Ritenour. *Radiation Protection in Medical Radiography*, 4th edn, Mosby, 2002. pp. 122–6.

8. A. False.
B. False: According to the recent amendment of ICRP June 2006 draft, gonads specific tissue weighting factor has decreased from 0.2 to 0.08. However, this is still classified as 'high risk'.
C. False.
D. False.
E. False.

Allisy-Roberts & Williams. *Farr's Physics for Medical Imaging*, 2nd edn, Saunders Elsevier, 2008. pp. 27–8.
Sherer, Visconti, and Ritenour. *Radiation Protection in Medical Radiography*, 4th edn, Mosby, 2002. pp. 122–6.

9. A. False: It is 0.012.
B. True.
C. False: It is 0.08.
D. True.
E. True.

Recommendations of the International Commission on Radiological Protection (www.icrp.org) http://www.icrp.org/docs/2005_recs_CONSULTATION_Draft1a.pdf

See Table 2.4 which summarizes organ- and tissue-specific weighting factors.

10. A. False: The unit for ESD is Gray (Gy).
B. False: The unit for Equivalent dose is Sieverts.
C. False: The unit for DAP is Gy cm^2.
D. True: Absorbed dose is measured in Gray and 1Gy = 1J/kg.
E. False: The unit for Effective dose is Sieverts.

11. A. True.
B. False: There is a threshold dose below which they do not occur.
C. False: They are dose dependent.
D. False: The threshold dose varies for different deterministic effects.
E. True.

Allisy-Roberts & Williams. *Farr's Physics for Medical Imaging*, 2nd edn, Saunders Elsevier, 2008. pp. 25–6.

12. A. False: The probability increases with increasing dose.
B. False: They occur after a latent period which lasts for many years.
C. True: They occur by chance and are not dose dependent but the chance of developing stochastic effects increases with the dose.
D. False.
E. True.

Allisy-Roberts & Williams. *Farr's Physics for Medical Imaging*, 2nd edn, Saunders Elsevier, 2008. pp. 26–7.

13. A. False.
B. True: Since the radiation weighting factor for both is one.
C. False: This is true for stochastic effects.
D. True.
E. False: It is a deterministic effect.

Allisy-Roberts & Williams. *Farr's Physics for Medical Imaging*, 2nd edn, Saunders Elsevier, 2008. pp. 25–7.

14. A. True.
B. True: Alpha particles have a large mass and double charge making them travel slowly through matter.
C. False: They are similar to helium nucleus with 2 protons and 2 neutrons.
D. False: Alpha particles are heavier.
E. False: They produce a large amount of ionization per unit length of the medium through which they travel making them unsafe for use in radiology.

15. A. True.
B. True.
C. True: The DRL is 3mGy.
D. False: Entrance surface dose is usually 5mGy. The DRL for an abdominal film is 7 mGy.
E. False: The skin dose rate of fluoroscopy is 5–50 mGy/min.

Allisy-Roberts & Williams. *Farr's Physics for Medical Imaging*, 2nd edn, Saunders Elsevier, 2008. p. 26.

16. A. True.
B. False: PA chest film—0.02 mSv.
C. False: CT chest typically—8 mSv.
D. True.
E. True.

Allisy-Roberts & Williams. *Farr's Physics for Medical Imaging*, 2nd edn, Saunders Elsevier, 2008. p. 44.

17. A. False.
B. False.
C. False.
D. True.
E. True.

Following exposure to ionizing radiation, chemical changes occur practically immediately (in seconds to minutes) and then molecular damage (in hours to decades).

Allisy-Roberts & Williams. *Farr's Physics for Medical Imaging*, 2nd edn, Saunders Elsevier, 2008. pp. 23–4.
Sherer, Visconti, and Ritenour. *Radiation Protection in Medical Radiography*, 4th edn, Mosby, 2002. pp. 105–55.

18. A. False.
B. False: Direct damage to tissue occurs by the rupture of covalent bonds and indirect damage by the production of free radicals.
C. True.
D. True.
E. False: It depends on the linear energy transfer of different ionizing radiations.

Allisy-Roberts & Williams. *Farr's Physics for Medical Imaging*, 2nd edn, Saunders Elsevier, 2008. pp. 23–4.
Sherer, Visconti, and Ritenour. *Radiation Protection in Medical Radiography*, 4th edn, Mosby, 2002. pp. 105–55.

Table 2.5 Entrance surface doses

Examination	Entrance Surface Dose (mGy) Typical Value	Entrance Surface Dose (mGy) National Diagnostic Reference Value (NDRL)
Skull	1.9	3
Chest PA	0.12	0.2
Lumbar spine AP	4.3	6
Lumbar spine lateral	10	14
Pelvis AP	3.2	4

Table 2.6 Typical effective doses

Investigation	Dose (mSV)
PA CXR	0.02
AP Pelvis	0.6
AXR	0.7
Lumbar Spine XR (2 films)	1
Barium Meal	2.5
IVU	3
Barium Enema	7
CT Brain	2
CT Chest	8
CT Abdomen	10–15
Tc-99m lung perfusion study	1
Tc-99m bone scan	4

19. A. True.
B. True.
C. True.
D. True.
E. True.

Allisy-Roberts & Williams. *Farr's Physics for Medical Imaging*, 2nd edn, Saunders Elsevier, 2008. pp. 26.

20. A. True.
B. True.
C. True.
D. True.
E. True.

Allisy-Roberts & Williams. *Farr's Physics for Medical Imaging*, 2nd edn, Saunders Elsevier, 2008. pp. 26–7.
Electronic Learning Database, E-Learning for Healthcare, Radiology—Integrated Training Initiative (R-ITI) – www.e-lfh.org.uk
Module: 8a_024: Biological Effects of Radiation Exposure on the Embryo, Fetus and Infant.

21. A. True: This is the period of organogenesis when the potential is highest.
B. True: A decrease in IQ is, however, seen up to the 25th week of pregnancy.
C. False: The pre-implantation phase poses the greatest risk of foetal death.
D. False: The risk is almost nil up to 3 weeks following which the risk remains for the rest of the pregnancy but is maximum in the first trimester.
E. True.

Electronic Learning Database, E-Learning for Healthcare, Radiology. Integrated Training Initiative (R-ITI) – www.e-lfh.org.uk
Module: 8a_024: Biological Effects of Radiation Exposure on the Embryo, Fetus and Infant.

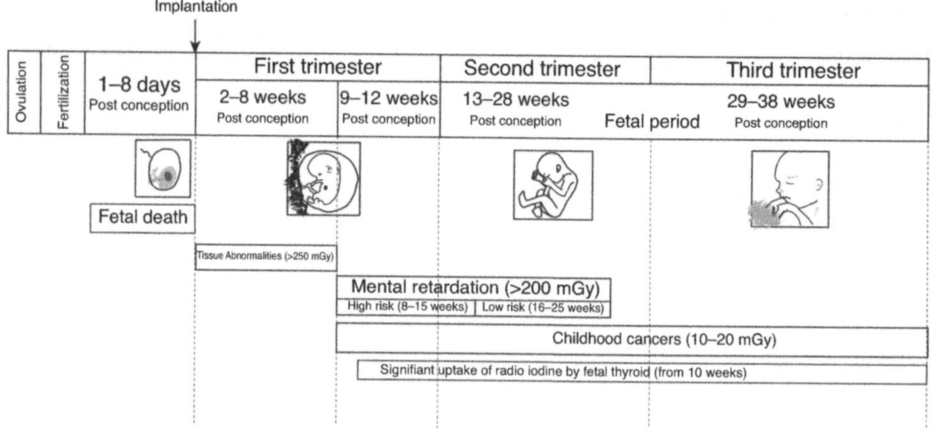

Figure 2.1 The effect of radiation on the foetus at various stages of development

22. A. False: It is 5% per Sv or 1 in 20,000 per mSv.
B. False: It is 3% per Gy or 1 in 33,000 per mGy.
C. False.
D. True.
E. False.

Sherer, Visconti, and Ritenour. *Radiation Protection in Medical Radiography*, 4th edn, Mosby, 2002. p. 107.

23. A. False: Potassium-40, a radioactive isotope of potassium is the commonest contributor of radiation from internal sources.
B. False: It is approximately 2.2 mSv per year.
C. True: Due to the presence of high amounts of radon the average dose received in Cornwall is approximately 7 mSv per year.
D. False: The decay of radon is primarily associated with the emission of alpha particles.
E. False: It is 370 μSv and accounts for 14% of the radiation from natural and artificial sources in the UK.

Allisy-Roberts & Williams. *Farr's Physics for Medical Imaging*, 2nd edn, Saunders Elsevier, 2008. pp. 28–9.

24. A. False: It requires an ionization chamber for measurement.
B. False.
C. True.
D. False.
E. True.

Allisy-Roberts & Williams. *Farr's Physics for Medical Imaging*, 2nd edn, Saunders Elsevier, 2008. pp. 17–19 and 45–6.

25. A. False: It is measured in Gray.
B. True: As this includes scatter.
C. True.
D. True.
E. True.

26. A. True.
B. False: The crystal is usually lithium fluoride.
C. True.
D. False: They cannot differentiate between radiation types.
E. False.

Allisy-Roberts & Williams. *Farr's Physics for Medical Imaging*, 2nd edn, Saunders Elsevier, 2008. pp. 36–7.
Electronic Learning Database, E-Learning for Healthcare, Radiology—Integrated Training Initiative (R-ITI) – www.e-lfh.org.uk
Module: 8a_005: Luminescence.
Module: 8a_052: Personal Dosimetry.

27. A. True.
B. False: The sensitivity is very similar to that of film.
C. True.
D. False.
E. True: As they can be made into various shapes, they can be used for the assessment of finger and eye doses.

Electronic Learning Database, E-Learning for Healthcare, Radiology—Integrated Training Initiative (R-ITI) – www.e-lfh.org.uk
Module: 8a_052: Personal Dosimetry.
Sherer, Visconti, and Ritenour. *Radiation Protection in Medical Radiography*, 4th edn, Mosby, 2002. pp. 225–32.

28. A. True.
B. False: A double-sided film emulsion is used.
C. False: They are subject to the environmental effects of heat, humidity, and chemical change.
D. False: A double-sided film emulsion is used but without a screen.
E. True.

Allisy-Roberts & Williams. *Farr's Physics for Medical Imaging*, 2nd edn, Saunders Elsevier, 2008. pp. 36–7.
Sherer, Visconti, and Ritenour. *Radiation Protection in Medical Radiography*, 4th edn, Mosby, 2002. pp. 225–32.

29. A. False.
B. False.
C. False.
D. True.
E. True.

Allisy-Roberts & Williams. *Farr's Physics for Medical Imaging*, 2nd edn, Saunders Elsevier, 2008. pp. 36–7.
Sherer, Visconti, and Ritenour. *Radiation Protection in Medical Radiography*, 4th edn, Mosby, 2002. pp. 225–32.

30. A. True.
B. False: They are relatively more expensive than film but can be reused.
C. False.
D. True: They can only read a dose once but TLDs can be re-used and read many times.
E. False: They are affected by environmental effects (especially heat).

Sherer, Visconti, and Ritenour. *Radiation Protection in Medical Radiography*, 4th edn, Mosby, 2002. pp. 225–32.

31. A. False.
B. False: TLDs are relative energy independent.
C. True.
D. True.
E. True.

32. A. True.
B. False.
C. True.
D. False: As they are subject to the environmental effects of heat, humidity, and chemical changes, they are unsuitable for monitoring over a period of 1 month.
E. False: It measures the absorbed dose, which we presume represents the whole body dose.

Sherer, Visconti, and Ritenour. *Radiation Protection in Medical Radiography*, 4th edn, Mosby, 2002. pp. 225–32.

33. A. False: Only electronic dosimeters have a precision better than 1%.
B. True.
C. True.
D. True.
E. False: The outer case is the cathode.

34. A. True.
B. True.
C. True.
D. False.
E. True.

Allisy-Roberts & Williams. *Farr's Physics for Medical Imaging*, 2nd edn, Saunders Elsevier, 2008. pp. 36–7.

35. A. True.
B. False: It must be worn under the lead apron.
C. True.
D. True: The holder has filters which are responsible for this function.
E. True: And 3% for high doses.

36. A. True.
B. False: They are used mainly in nuclear medicine to detect contamination.
C. True.
D. False: They can detect all types of radiation but cannot distinguish them.
E. False: The central wire is the anode.

Electronic Learning Database, E-Learning for Healthcare, Radiology—Integrated Training Initiative (R-ITI) – www.e-lfh.org.uk
Module: 8a_050: Radiation Detectors.

chapter

3

IRR (99) AND IRMER (2000)

QUESTIONS

1. Regarding controlled areas:

A. Are required where a person working is likely to receive an effective dose more than 3 mSv per year.
B. Are required where a person working is likely to receive a radiation dose greater than three-tenths of any dose limit.
C. Are required where the external dose rate could exceed 5μSv per hour averaged over the working day.
D. An intervention suite is an example.
E. The injection room used for radionuclide imaging must be designated a controlled area.

2. Controlled areas:

A. Are required where a person working is likely to receive an equivalent dose more than 6mSv per year.
B. May be required where there is a risk of radioactive contamination.
C. Must be described in the local rules.
D. Are permitted areas for pregnant staff.
E. Are monitored by the Radiation Protection Advisor.

3. Supervised areas:

A. Are required only where a person working is likely to receive an effective dose more than 3mSv per year.
B. Are required only where a person working there is likely to receive a radiation dose greater than three-tenths of any dose limit.
C. The waiting room for patients who have been injected with a radiopharmaceutical is an example.
D. Must be clearly marked with warning signs.
E. Can become a controlled area.

4. Regarding IRR 99:

A. The employer must consult a Radiation Protection Supervisor prior to installing new equipment.
B. The Healthcare Commission must be informed of the use of ionizing radiation by the employer.
C. The Radiation Protection Supervisor (RPS) is invariably a medical physics expert.
D. The Radiation Protection Supervisor (RPS) must be an employee of the organization.
E. *Critical examination* of equipment is the responsibility of the employer.

5. Regarding IRR 99:

A. The regulations govern the safety of staff, patients, and public.
B. The Health and Safety Executive is the governing authority.
C. The local rules should include descriptions of all designated areas.
D. The equivalent dose limits are concerned with stochastic effects.
E. The effective dose limits are designed to prevent deterministic effects.

6. The following annual dose limits apply:

A. The equivalent dose to the lens of the eye of an employee is 500mSv.
B. The effective dose to a member of public is 2mSv.
C. The equivalent dose to the skin of an employee is 500mSv.
D. The dose to the abdomen of a woman of reproductive age should not be more than 13mSv in any consecutive 3-month period.
E. The equivalent dose to the extremities of an employee is 150mSv.

7. The following annual dose limits apply:

A. The equivalent dose to the skin of a member of the public is 50mSv.
B. The foetus of a pregnant employee should not receive more than 0.1mSv.
C. The equivalent dose to the lens of a member of the public is 15mSv.
D. The equivalent dose to the extremities of a member of the public is 150mSv.
E. The effective dose to an employee is 10mSv.

8. IRR 99 states that the following people may enter controlled areas:

A. Classified employees.
B. Radiographers.
C. Non-classified employees entering under a written agreement.
D. Patients having radionuclide imaging.
E. Operators.

9. Controlled areas:

A. Non-classified workers are not permitted to enter controlled areas.
B. Require special working procedures to restrict exposure.
C. Access to radiology staff to controlled areas must be restricted.
D. Are needed for portable x-ray units.
E. Must be clearly marked with warning signs and indicate the nature of the source and risk.

10. The following events must be reported if a patient receives:

A. 15 times the intended dose for a chest x-ray.
B. 8 times the intended dose for a mammogram.
C. 10 times the intended dose for a lumbar spine x-ray.
D. 1.5 times the intended dose for a CT abdomen.
E. Twice the intended dose for a barium enema.

11. The following events must be reported to the HSE:

A. A patient receives a greater than intended dose because of an operator fault.
B. A patient receives 1.6 times the intended dose for an angiogram.
C. Loss of radioactive material.
D. Spillage of any amount of radioactive material.
E. A patient receives 1.3 times the intended dose during radionuclide therapy.

12. According to IRR 99:

A. The RPA is responsible for quality assurance.
B. The RPS is responsible for designation of radiation areas.
C. The RPA must be an employee of the organization.
D. The RPA is responsible for supervising staff dose monitoring.
E. The RPS must be consulted prior to the installation of new x-ray equipment.

13. Regarding classified workers:

A. The annual effective dose limit is 6mSv.
B. An employee above the age of 16 years can be classified.
C. The records of classified workers must be kept for 25 years beyond the date that the individual stops working as a classified personnel.
D. They must undergo annual health checks.
E. Staff working in nuclear medicine are classified workers.

14. Regarding standards for x-ray equipment:

A. Leakage radiation from the tube must be less than 1mGy/hr at 1 metre from the focus.
B. For portable x-ray equipment the total filtration of the tube and its assembly should not be less than 1.5mm of aluminium.
C. For fluoroscopy equipment the collimators should be capable of restricting the field size down to $2.5 \times 2.5\text{cm}^2$.
D. Skin entrance dose rates for fluoroscopy should not exceed 100mGy/min.
E. For mobile x-ray equipment the position of the exposure switch should be designed such that the operator can stand at least 1m from the tube and x-ray beam.

15. Regarding Quality Assurance:

A. The installer or RPA can complete the critical examination of new equipment.
B. Tests on all equipment, annually at least, are mandatory.
C. Requires the equipment used for testing to be calibrated.
D. Is not a requirement under IRMER 2000.
E. Is a requirement under IRR 99.

16. Regarding dose limits and dose constraint:

A. Dose limits do not apply to patients.
B. National rules apply for comforters and carers of patients.
C. The dose limits can be relaxed for comforters and carers.
D. A dose constraint is a dose limit of radiation.
E. The relaxation of dose limits can routinely be applied to employees.

17. According to IRR 99:

A. A radiation dose of 30mSv in a single year may be acceptable to a classified worker.
B. A classified worker is one whose radiation dose is likely to exceed one-tenths of any dose limit.
C. The RPA is responsible for the review of local rules.
D. The RPA can carry out critical examination of equipment.
E. An x-ray department can have more than one Radiation Protection Supervisor.

18. Under IRR 99:

A. The annual effective dose limit for a trainee employee under the age of 18 years is 6mSv.
B. The annual equivalent dose limit to the lens of the eye of a trainee employee under the age of 18 years is 150mSv.
C. The RPA may also be a medical physics expert.
D. The RPS is responsible for ensuring monitoring equipment is calibrated.
E. To work as a classified person the individual must be certified as being medically fit to work prior to employment.

19. An effective dose of 6mSv:

A. Carries a risk of about 1 in 3000 of a fatal cancer.
B. Would be excessive for a barium enema examination.
C. Is the annual dose limit for a trainee classified worker.
D. Is approximately 5 times the annual background radiation dose in the UK.
E. Is approximately 10 times the effective dose of an AP pelvis radiograph.

20. Concerning IRR 99:

A. The dose limits depend on the weighting factor of the radiation type to which the person is exposed.
B. The annual dose limits for comforters and carers is 3mSv.
C. The RPA must be present in the x-ray department during working hours.
D. The aim is to ensure that the radiation dose to employees and public is as low as reasonably achievable.
E. The regulations do not apply to radiation therapy.

21. Under IRMER 2000:

A. It is binding on the employer to identify the referrer.
B. Only doctors and dentists may act as referrers.
C. Radiographers can perform the role of practitioners.
D. The employer is responsible for ensuring patient doses are as low as reasonably practicable (ALARP).
E. A referrer is not liable for prosecution.

22. Regarding Diagnostic Reference Levels (DRLs):

A. Can be different for the same examination in different hospitals.
B. An investigation must be initiated if a patient DRL has been exceeded.
C. A DRL should be expressed as entrance surface dose.
D. Local DRLs cannot be higher than national levels.
E. The national DRL for a chest PA radiograph is 0.2mGy (ESD).

23. The following are true under IRMER 2000:

A. The operator is responsible for justification of an exposure.
B. It does not apply to individuals participating voluntarily in a research programme.
C. It does not apply to individuals for pre-employment occupational health assessment.
D. Referrers need to be trained adequately for requesting radiological investigations.
E. Preparation of a radiopharmaceutical is the responsibility of the operator.

24. The following statements regarding IRMER 2000 are true:

A. The operator must be a registered healthcare professional.
B. A radiographer can justify and authorize an exposure.
C. Cardiologists cannot perform the role of practitioners.
D. Only a practitioner can authorize an exposure.
E. Only a practitioner can justify an exposure.

25. The following are true of IRR 99:

A. It is mandatory to monitor doses of persons working with radiation.
B. In conjunction with the employer the RPS investigates overexposures.
C. The employer is responsible for the training of employees.
D. Does not allow a trainee below the age of 18 years in supervised and controlled areas.
E. The radiation dose records of classified workers need to be submitted to HSE certified dose record keeping authorities.

26. Regarding radiation legislation:

A. MARS 1978 is responsible for the storage and disposal of radioactive substances.
B. The organization must hold an ARSAC (Administration of Radioactive Substances Advisory Committee) certificate to carry out nuclear medicine investigations.
C. An ARSAC certificate needs to be renewed every 3 years.
D. IRMER requires that the employee ensure that personal protective equipment is properly used.
E. RSA 1993 is concerned with the protection of the population and environment.

27. The following statements are true:

A. A radioactive substance can only be administered by an ARSAC certificate holder.
B. The annual whole body dose for cardiologists is usually higher than for radiologists.
C. From working in a radiology department most staff receive < 1mSv annual radiation.
D. The HSE must be notified if a non-classified member of staff receives >6mSv in a 3-month period.
E. DRLs for CT scanning are generally in terms of Computed Tomography Dose Index (CTDI).

28. The following statements are true:

A. The principle of optimization is that the benefit from radiation exceeds the risks.
B. Following radionuclide imaging a lactating mother must interrupt breast feeding for 5 days.
C. A pregnant patient cannot have radionuclide imaging.
D. Optimization includes quality assurance programmes to ensure equipment performance.
E. The HSE must be notified if the wrong patient has undergone an investigation.

29. Concerning radiation protection:

A. Females between the ages of 14 and 55 years being exposed to ionizing radiation must be asked about the possibility of pregnancy.
B. Providing post procedure information to patients who have undergone a nuclear medicine investigation comes under the domain of optimization.
C. Radiation weighting factors are measured in Gray.
D. Lead aprons used in interventional radiology are generally 0.35mm lead equivalent.
E. 12mm of barium will provide the same protection as 1mm of lead.

30. Concerning radiation protection of staff and patients:

A. 2.5mm lead equivalent filter should be used for routine radiological procedures.
B. Lead screen panels used in x-ray rooms to protect staff are usually 5mm thick.
C. In fluoroscopy, the scattered radiation to staff from an overcouch tube is less than an undercouch one.
D. Thyroid collars used in radiology have 0.5mm lead equivalence.
E. For chest radiography, the film to focus distance should not be less than 30cm.

31. The following are true:

A. A 0.25mm lead apron transmits less than 3% of the radiation.
B. The average daily dose from natural background radiation is 6μSv.
C. The radiation dose rate from air travel is about 2μSv/hr.
D. A radiologist wearing a lead apron is adequately protected from the primary radiation.
E. The Environment Agency is the enforcing authority for the Radioactive Substances Act 1993.

chapter 3

IRR (99) AND IRMER (2000)

ANSWERS

1. A. False: Are required where a person working receives more than 6mSv per year.
B. True.
C. False: Are required where the external dose rate could exceed 7.5μSv per hour.
D. True.
E. False: Designation of the injection room as a controlled area depends on the nature, dose, and risk of contamination of the radioactive materials used. This is decided at a prior risk assessment by the radiation protection adviser (RPA), and although not always necessary it generally is designated as a controlled area.

Allisy-Roberts & Williams. *Farr's Physics for Medical Imaging*, 2nd edn, Saunders Elsevier, 2008. p. 33. Sherer, Visconti, and Ritenour. *Radiation Protection in Medical Radiography*, 4th edn, Mosby, 2002. pp. 202–3.

2. A. False: Are required where a person working receives an effective dose more than 6mSv per year.
B. True.
C. True.
D. True: Generally it is not advisable. However, if risk assessment deems it appropriate then pregnant staff can work in controlled areas under this condition (nb. think of pregnant radiographers).
E. False: This is the responsibility of the Radiation Protection Supervisor.

Allisy-Roberts & Williams. *Farr's Physics for Medical Imaging*, 2nd edn, Saunders Elsevier, 2008. p. 33.

3. A. False: Are required where a person working could exceed the dose limit for a member of the public (1mSv per year).
B. False: They are required where a person working is likely to receive a radiation dose greater than one-tenths of any dose limit.
C. True.
D. True.
E. True: If the dose limits are exceeded and should be monitored regularly.

Allisy-Roberts & Williams. *Farr's Physics for Medical Imaging*, 2nd edn, Saunders Elsevier, 2008. p. 33.

4. A. False: The Radiation Protection Advisor must be consulted.
B. False: The employer must notify the Health and Safety Executive (HSE).
C. False: Any suitably trained staff member, e.g. radiographer, can take up the role of RPS.
D. True.
E. False: It is the responsibility of the installer.

Allisy-Roberts & Williams. *Farr's Physics for Medical Imaging*, 2nd edn, Saunders Elsevier, 2008. p. 34.
Electronic Learning Database, E-Learning for Healthcare, Radiology—Integrated Training Initiative (R-ITI) – www.e-lfh.org.uk
Module: 8a_032: IRR99

5. A. False: The regulations govern the safety of staff and public but not patients.
B. True.
C. True.
D. False: Equivalent dose limits are designed to ensure doses are kept below the threshold doses for deterministic effects.
E. False: The effective dose limit is concerned with stochastic risk.

Allisy-Roberts & Williams. *Farr's Physics for Medical Imaging*, 2nd edn, Saunders Elsevier, 2008. pp. 31–3.

6. A. False.
B. False.
C. True.
D. True.
E. False.

Allisy-Roberts & Williams. *Farr's Physics for Medical Imaging*, 2nd edn, Saunders Elsevier, 2008. p. 32.

7. A. True.
B. False: A dose constraint of 1mSv is applied as the foetus is regarded as a member of the public.
C. True.
D. False.
E. False.

Allisy-Roberts & Williams. *Farr's Physics for Medical Imaging*, 2nd edn, Saunders Elsevier, 2008. p. 32.

8. A. True.
B. False: Please see Figures 3.1 aand 3.2.
C. True.
D. True.
E. False.

Electronic Learning Database, E-Learning for Healthcare, Radiology—Integrated Training Initiative (R-ITI) – www.e-lfh.org.uk
Module: 8a_032: IRR99

9. A. False: Local rules may allow non-classified workers to enter a controlled area.
B. True.
C. True.
D. True: This normally extends within 2m of the x-ray tube and patient.
E. True.

Allisy-Roberts & Williams. *Farr's Physics for Medical Imaging*, 2nd edn, Saunders Elsevier, 2008. p. 33.

10. A. False.
B. False.
C. True.
D. True.
E. True.

Allisy-Roberts & Williams. *Farr's Physics for Medical Imaging*, 2nd edn, Saunders Elsevier, 2008. p. 38.

11. A. False: HSE needs to be informed of events secondary to equipment faults; those due to operator errors need to be reported to the Care Quality Commission, previously known as the Healthcare Commission.
B. True.
C. True.
D. False: Only spillage causing significant contamination needs to be reported.
E. False.

12. A. False: The employer is responsible for quality assurance.
B. False: This is the responsibility of the RPA.
C. False: He or she can be an external consultant.
D. False: This is the responsibility of the RPS.
E. False: The RPA must be consulted.

Allisy-Roberts & Williams. *Farr's Physics for Medical Imaging*, 2nd edn, Saunders Elsevier, 2008. p. 34.

Learning Points

Table 3.1 Annual dose limits

Dose Limits	**Classified workers age > 18**	**Non-classified workers**	**Others**
Effective dose (mSv)	20	6	1
Equivalent dose to the lens of the eye (mSv)	150	50	15
Equivalent dose to an extremity (mSv)	500	150	50
Equivalent dose to the skin (mSv)	500	150	50

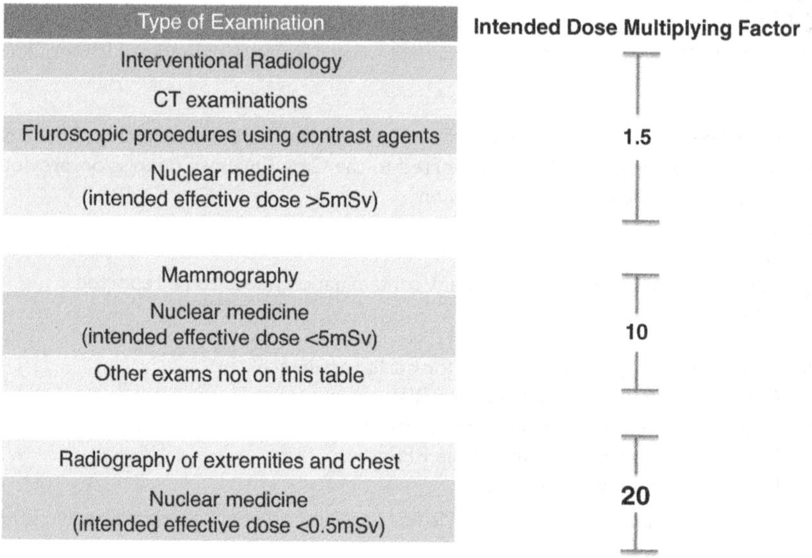

Type of Examination	**Intended Dose Multiplying Factor**
Interventional Radiology CT examinations Fluroscopic procedures using contrast agents Nuclear medicine (intended effective dose >5mSv)	1.5
Mammography Nuclear medicine (intended effective dose <5mSv) Other exams not on this table	10
Radiography of extremities and chest Nuclear medicine (intended effective dose <0.5mSv)	20

Figure 3.1 HSE guide concerning patient overexposures involving radiation equipment

13. A. False: This is the annual effective dose limit for non-classified workers, that for classified is 20mSv.
B. False: To be classified the individual must be 18 years old or over.
C. False: The records must be kept for 50 years after the individual stops working or until the individual is 75 years of age.
D. True.
E. False: Staff working in nuclear medicine are very rarely required to be classified.

Allisy-Roberts & Williams. *Farr's Physics for Medical Imaging*, 2nd edn, Saunders Elsevier, 2008. pp. 34–7.

14. A. True.
B. False: It should be not less than 2.5mm of aluminium.
C. False: They should be capable of restricting the field size down to 5 × 5cm^2.
D. True.
E. False: It must be at least 2m.

Allisy-Roberts & Williams. *Farr's Physics for Medical Imaging*, 2nd edn, Saunders Elsevier, 2008. p. 35.
Sherer, Visconti, and Ritenour. *Radiation Protection in Medical Radiography*, 4th edn, Mosby, 2002. pp. 206–23.

15. A. True: Though it is the responsibility of the installer it can be completed by either and ideally the installer must involve RPA.
B. False.
C. True.
D. False.
E. True.

Allisy-Roberts & Williams. *Farr's Physics for Medical Imaging*, 2nd edn, Saunders Elsevier, 2008. p. 36.

16. A. True.
B. False: Local rules are to be applied depending on the individual case but IRR99 does specify limits.
C. True.
D. False: A constraint is a maximum which may be exceeded.
E. False: They can be relaxed only in cases of emergencies.

Allisy-Roberts & Williams. *Farr's Physics for Medical Imaging*, 2nd edn, Saunders Elsevier, 2008. p. 32.

17. A. True: As long as the dose received by the individual does not exceed 100mSv over 5 years.
B. False: A classified worker is one whose radiation dose is likely to exceed three-tenths of any dose limit.
C. False: This is the responsibility of the Radiation Protection Supervisor.
D. True.
E. True.

Electronic Learning Database, E-Learning for Healthcare, Radiology—Integrated Training Initiative (R-ITI) – www.e-lfh.org.uk
Module: 8a_032: IRR99

18. A. True.
B. False: The dose limit is 50mSv.
C. True.
D. False: This is the responsibility of the RPA.
E. True.

Electronic Learning Database, E-Learning for Healthcare, Radiology—Integrated Training Initiative (R-ITI) – www.e-lfh.org.uk
Module: 8a_032: IRR99

19. A. True: The risk of fatal cancer is 1 in 20,000 per mSv making the risk from 6mSv about 1 in 3,000.
B. False: The typical effective dose from a barium enema examination is 7mSv.
C. False: The annual dose limit for trainees is 6mSv, but trainees cannot be classified.
D. False: The annual background radiation dose in the UK is 2.2mSv making 6mSv roughly 3 times the annual background radiation dose in the UK.
E. True: The typical effective dose of an AP pelvis radiograph is 0.6mSv.

Electronic Learning Database, E-Learning for Healthcare, Radiology—Integrated Training Initiative (R-ITI) – www.e-lfh.org.uk
Module: 8a_030: Principles of Radiation Protection

20. A. False: The doses are in terms of equivalent or effective doses, hence the weighting factor of the type of radiation has already been accounted for.
B. False: There are no dose limits for comforters and carers but IRR recommends that the employer set a dose constraint for these situations.
C. False: The RPA is often an external consultant and need not be present at all times.
D. False: The IRR is governed by the principle of as low as reasonably practicable (ALARP).
E. False.

21. A. True.
B. False: Nurse practitioners and physiotherapists may act as referrers (but must be state registered).
C. True.
D. True.
E. False: He or she can be prosecuted if adequate clinical information or the pregnancy status of the patient is not provided.

Allisy-Roberts & Williams. *Farr's Physics for Medical Imaging*, 2nd edn, Saunders Elsevier, 2008. pp. 38–9.
Electronic Learning Database, E-Learning for Healthcare, Radiology—Integrated Training Initiative (R-ITI) – www.e-lfh.org.uk
Module: 8a_033a-c: IRMER

22. A. True.
B. False: DRLs are not dose limits but guidance for dose levels for typical examinations in standard-sized patients.
C. False: They can be expressed as DAP, kv, mAs, screening time, etc.
D. False: They can be higher if justified on clinical grounds.
E. True.

Allisy-Roberts & Williams. *Farr's Physics for Medical Imaging*, 2nd edn, Saunders Elsevier, 2008. pp. 39–40.

23. A. False: The practitioner justifies an exposure.
B. False.
C. False.
D. False: Training is mandatory only for practitioners and operators.
E. True.

Allisy-Roberts & Williams. *Farr's Physics for Medical Imaging*, 2nd edn, Saunders Elsevier, 2008. pp. 38–9.
Electronic Learning Database, E-Learning for Healthcare, Radiology—Integrated Training Initiative (R-ITI) – www.e-lfh.org.uk
Module: 8a_033a-c: IRMER

24. A. False: The medical physics expert or service engineer to an x-ray machine can be an operator.
B. True.
C. False: They are practitioners in respect to cardiac intervention studies.
D. False: Under written justification guidelines from the practitioner, an operator may authorize examinations.
E. True.

Allisy-Roberts & Williams. *Farr's Physics for Medical Imaging*, 2nd edn, Saunders Elsevier, 2008. pp. 38–9.

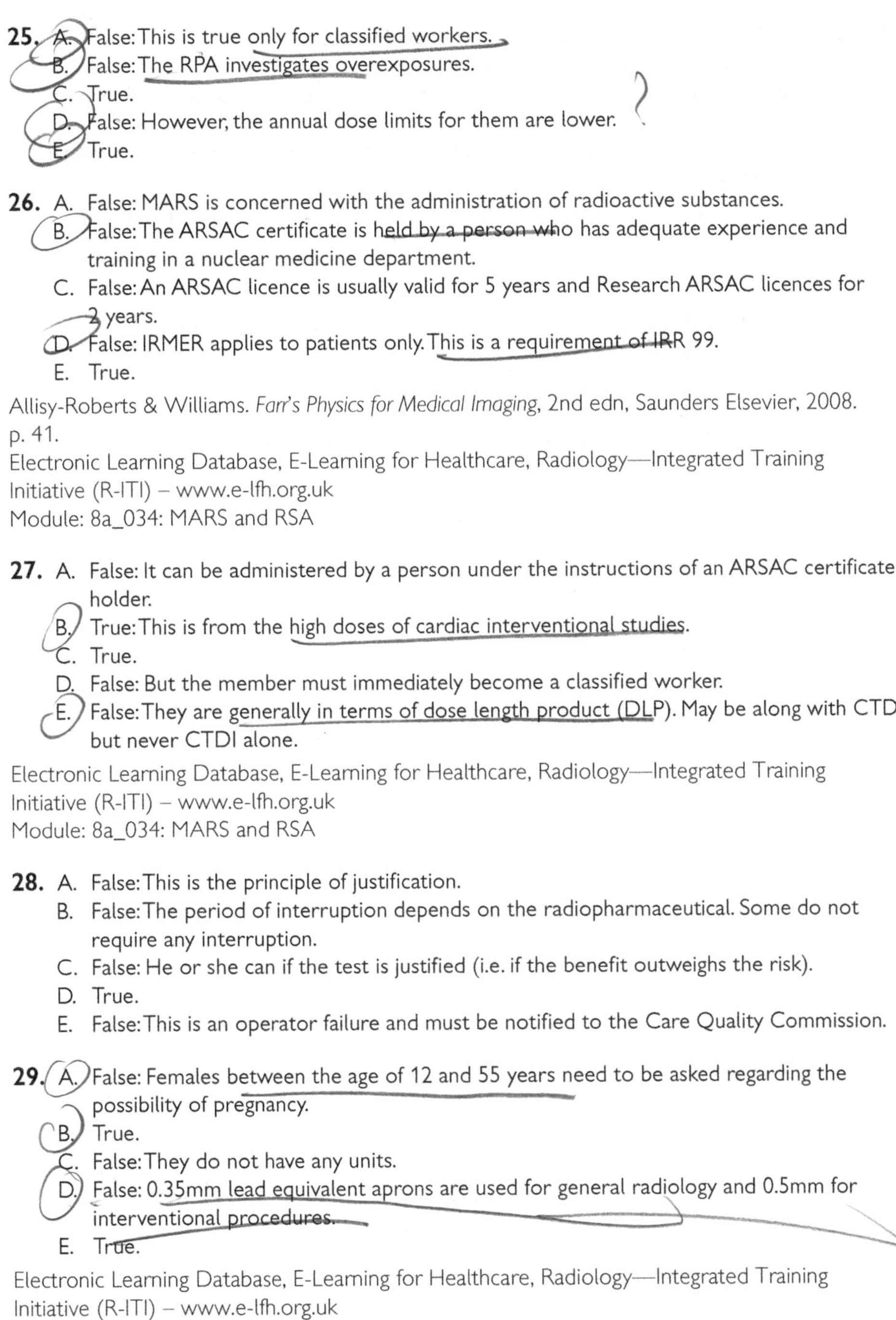

25. A. False: This is true only for classified workers.
B. False: The RPA investigates overexposures.
C. True.
D. False: However, the annual dose limits for them are lower.
E. True.

26. A. False: MARS is concerned with the administration of radioactive substances.
B. False: The ARSAC certificate is held by a person who has adequate experience and training in a nuclear medicine department.
C. False: An ARSAC licence is usually valid for 5 years and Research ARSAC licences for 2 years.
D. False: IRMER applies to patients only. This is a requirement of IRR 99.
E. True.

Allisy-Roberts & Williams. *Farr's Physics for Medical Imaging*, 2nd edn, Saunders Elsevier, 2008. p. 41.
Electronic Learning Database, E-Learning for Healthcare, Radiology—Integrated Training Initiative (R-ITI) – www.e-lfh.org.uk
Module: 8a_034: MARS and RSA

27. A. False: It can be administered by a person under the instructions of an ARSAC certificate holder.
B. True: This is from the high doses of cardiac interventional studies.
C. True.
D. False: But the member must immediately become a classified worker.
E. False: They are generally in terms of dose length product (DLP). May be along with CTDI but never CTDI alone.

Electronic Learning Database, E-Learning for Healthcare, Radiology—Integrated Training Initiative (R-ITI) – www.e-lfh.org.uk
Module: 8a_034: MARS and RSA

28. A. False: This is the principle of justification.
B. False: The period of interruption depends on the radiopharmaceutical. Some do not require any interruption.
C. False: He or she can if the test is justified (i.e. if the benefit outweighs the risk).
D. True.
E. False: This is an operator failure and must be notified to the Care Quality Commission.

29. A. False: Females between the age of 12 and 55 years need to be asked regarding the possibility of pregnancy.
B. True.
C. False: They do not have any units.
D. False: 0.35mm lead equivalent aprons are used for general radiology and 0.5mm for interventional procedures.
E. True.

Electronic Learning Database, E-Learning for Healthcare, Radiology—Integrated Training Initiative (R-ITI) – www.e-lfh.org.uk
Module: 8a_042: Protection of the Patient in Diagnostic Radiology

30. A. False: 2.5mm aluminium equivalent filter should be used.
B. False: They are usually made of 2mm lead.
C. False: The radiation from an overcouch tube is more than for an undercouch one.
D. True.
E. False: It should not be less than 60cm for fixed equipment. 30cm may be permissible for portable units.

Allisy-Roberts & Williams. *Farr's Physics for Medical Imaging*, 2nd edn, Saunders Elsevier, 2008. pp. 41–4.

See Figure 3.2.

31. A. False: 0.25, 0.35, and 0.5mm lead equivalent aprons transmit approximately 5%, 3%, and 1.5% of radiation respectively.
B. True.
C. False: It is about 4μSv/hr.
D. False: Lead aprons provide protection only from scattered radiation.
E. True.

Learning Points

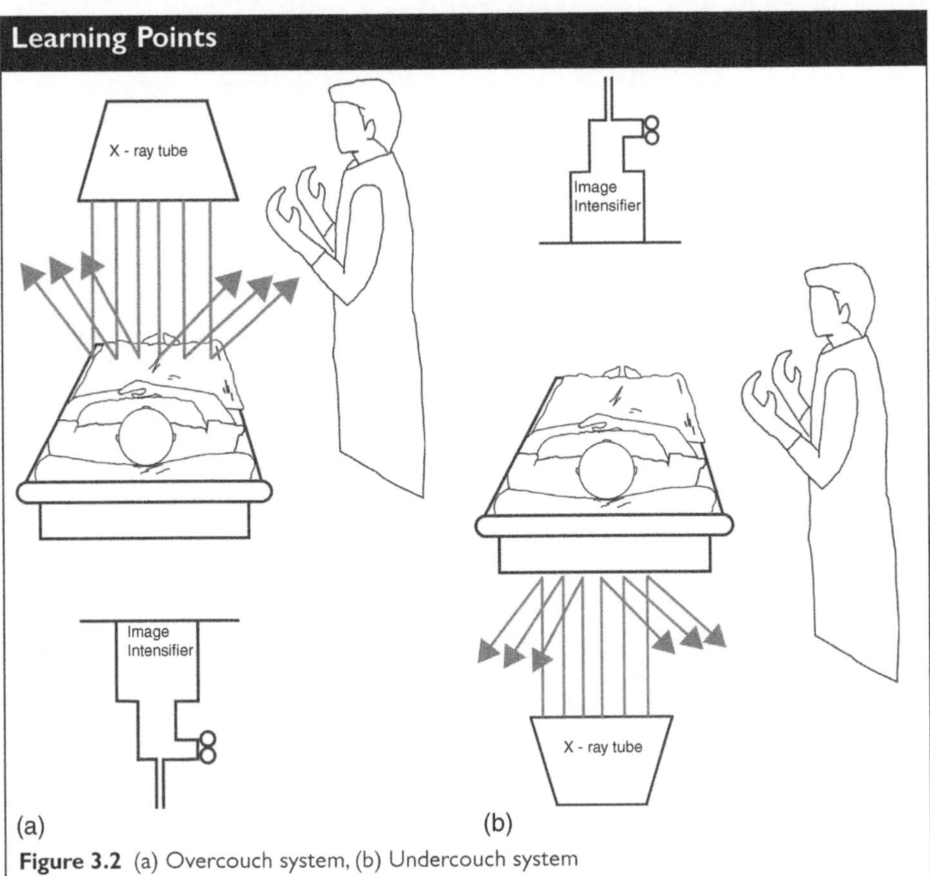

Figure 3.2 (a) Overcouch system, (b) Undercouch system

chapter

4

IMAGE QUALITY AND X-RAY PRODUCTION

QUESTIONS

1. Regarding the interaction of radiation with the body:

A. Photons of energy of 40keV react with soft tissues of the body, predominantly by the Compton reaction.
B. Bone has a higher effective atomic number than soft tissue for a diagnostic energy range.
C. For a given energy and medium in the diagnostic range the actual linear attenuation coefficient is always higher than the Compton linear attenuation coefficient.
D. The units of the mass energy absorption coefficient are centimetres (squared)/kg.
E. The linear attenuation coefficient is the mass attenuation coefficient divided by the density.

2. Regarding x-ray production:

A. Beam quality depends on kV and voltage waveform.
B. Beam intensity depends on the atomic number of the target, tube current, kV, and kV waveform.
C. Characteristic radiation constitutes a steadily increasing proportion of the total with increasing kV.
D. No characteristic K shell radiation is produced from a Tungsten target at kVp 65.
E. After 2.5mm of aluminium filtration, the peak intensity of an x-ray beam occurs about 1/3 of the maximum kVp.

3. Regarding attenuation for an x-ray beam:

A. For a monochromatic beam attenuation is exponential.
B. The amount of attenuation increases as electron density increases.
C. Throughout the range of 20–100keV a greater proportion of interactions are photoelectric for soft tissue as compared to bone.
D. The unit of mass attenuation coefficient (MAC) is grams per cm squared.
E. The half value thickness is the thickness of a substance that will reduce the intensity of a beam by 50%.

4. The mass attenuation coefficient:

A. Is defined as the linear attenuation coefficient (LAC) divided by the density.
B. Is affected by the atomic number.
C. Is directly proportional to the half value layer (HVL).
D. Is inversely proportional to the radiation energy.
E. Depends on the type of radiation interaction.

5. Concerning the Compton effect:

A. There is interaction between a free electron and a photon
B. For incident photons of equal energy, more energy is lost from the photon as the scatter angle increases.
C. High energy radiation undergoes more scattering events than lower energy radiation.
D. The amount of scattering that occurs depends on the electron density of the scattering material.
E. The larger the angle through which the photon is scattered, the more energy it loses.

6. Compton interactions tend to reduce the contrast in the image because:

A. The mean photon energy is reduced.
B. The recoil electrons affect the image.
C. The photon undergoes a change in direction.
D. Attenuation of the beam is increased.
E. Compton interactions in the screen reduce contrast.

7. Scattered radiation reaching the film would be expected to be reduced by:

A. A high tube kV.
B. A moving grid.
C. Coning.
D. Using tubes with higher heat rating.
E. Placing a thin sheet of zinc on the film cassette.

8. Concerning anti-scatter grids:

A. With a parallel grid, cut-off limits the maximum field size.
B. With a focused grid, cut-off limits the range of focus to film distance.
C. A linear grid reduces contrast in the direction perpendicular to the lead strips.
D. Use of a grid may increase patient dose by a factor of 4.
E. Grid lines in an image occur only if a stationary grid is used.

9. In the use of grids:

A. The interspaces may be filled with aluminium.
B. The grid ratio is defined as the ratio between the height of the lead strips and the distance between them.
C. The interspaces are usually much thicker than the lead strips.
D. In the linear grid it may be possible for the x-ray tube to be angled without the effect of 'grid cut-off'.
E. A crossed grid is made of two superimposed linear grids having different focusing distances.

10. Use of a grid normally leads to:

A. Reduced scatter dose to the patient.
B. An increase in the exposure latitude of the film screen combination.
C. An increase in the exposure to the patient.
D. A higher mean energy of the beam reaching the film.
E. A reduction of scatter radiation reaching the film.

11. A focused grid:

A. May cause radiation cut-off at large field sizes.
B. Should be used within a defined range of focus to film distance.
C. Requires an increase in patient dose to achieve the same film density as an exposure without a grid.
D. Reduces geometric distortion of the image.
E. Improves contrast by reducing the amount of scattered radiation reaching the film.

12. X-ray exposure to the patient may be reduced by:

A. Adding a 2mm aluminium filter to the beam.
B. Using a higher kVp.
C. Reducing the x-ray target–object distance.
D. Using rare earth screens.
E. Using a Potter-Bucky grid.

13. Secondary radiation grids:

A. Usual grid ratio is 4:1–16:1.
B. As grid height increases, resolution of the image improves.
C. Grid factor is the ratio of incident radiation to transmitted radiation.
D. They absorb both primary and secondary radiation.
E. Grid ratio is the ability of the grid to stop primary radiation.

14. The focal spot of the x-ray tube:

A. Is the cause of the penumbra on the image.
B. Focal spot motion causes motion unsharpness.
C. Causes absorption unsharpness.
D. Emits radiation of uniform intensity across its face.
E. Significantly influences the degree of magnification of objects about the size of the focal spot.

15. Regarding the focal spot:

A. Its size increases with an increase in the tube current.
B. Its resolving capacity can be measured by pinhole imaging.
C. Its size increases with increased kVp.
D. The focal spot is shorter when measured at the cathode end than at the anode end.
E. A focal spot has improved resolving power if it has a centrally peaked radiation intensity distribution.

16. The effective focal spot is governed by:

A. The target angle.
B. The target size.
C. The line focus principle.
D. The filament size.
E. The applied kV.

17. Concerning the 'air-gap' technique:

A. Scatter is removed from the beam.
B. An air gap of more than 30cm is needed.
C. This technique is equivalent to using a grid, but a higher patient dose is needed.
D. Grids are used in preference to an air-gap technique when imaging paediatric patients.
E. An air gap requires increased patient dose.

18. Regarding tomography:

A. The x-ray tube and cassette move in opposite directions.
B. A large swing angle gives a thicker slice.
C. Blurring is used as an advantage.
D. This technique is often used in intravenous urography.
E. Increasing focus–film distance increases slice thickness.

19. In tomography:

A. The contrast is dependent on the slice thickness.
B. Only structures at right angles to the film appear sharp.
C. Tomography is most useful when imaging structures with low inherent contrast.
D. Image unsharpness is unaffected by the use of tomography.
E. Patient dose is higher than in conventional radiography.

20. When using a narrow angle in tomography:

A. The section thickness increases.
B. Tissue contrast is reduced.
C. The blurring of structures outside the focal plane is increased.
D. The unsharpness within the focal plane is increased.
E. The tendency for phantom image formation increases.

21. In an x-ray tube, a rotating anode:

A. Results in a larger focal spot.
B. Increases the maximum tube rating.
C. Allows larger exposures to be made when compared with a stationary anode.
D. Reduces heat input to the x-ray tube.
E. Is constructed from molybdenum with a tungsten target.

22. In a rotating anode x-ray tube:

A. The anode stem is made of tungsten.
B. The effective focal spot size depends on the anode angle.
C. Heat is removed from the anode mainly by thermal conduction.
D. Heat is removed more efficiently when a low current is used.
E. The anode heel effect occurs in a direction parallel to the anode–cathode axis.

23. Filtration of the x-ray beam:

A. In the patient is known as inherent filtration.
B. Tends to increase tissue contrast.
C. Aluminium is more efficient than copper for filtering off higher energy radiation.
D. Would be expected to decrease the maximum photon energy.
E. Helps to decrease the amount of loading on the x-ray tube.

24. Inherent filtration:

A. The glass envelope is responsible for most of it.
B. It varies approximately between 0.5 and 1mm of aluminium equivalent.
C. Decreases tissue contrast.
D. Beryllium has an atomic number of less than 10.
E. It includes the oil surrounding the tube.

25. In the x-ray tube:

A. The effective focal spot used in fluoroscopy is usually less than 1mm.
B. The intensity of the x-ray beam is greatest when perpendicular to the incident electron beam.
C. Rotating anodes help in heat dissipation.
D. A tungsten-rhenium alloy does not roughen with use as much as a pure tungsten anode.
E. The thermal rating of the tube increases as the kV is increased.

26. The maximum photon energy in the spectrum of x-rays from an x-ray set is influenced by:

A. The peak tube potential (kV).
B. Filtration.
C. Tube current (mA).
D. Target material.
E. The tube potential waveform.

27. If on taking an x-ray, the exposure (mAs) is set to keep the film density constant, then:

A. An increase in tube potential (kV) will reduce the effective dose to the patient.
B. Using a faster film screen combination will reduce the effective dose to the patient.
C. Selecting a smaller focal spot will not affect the patient dose.
D. Increasing the x-ray field size will increase effective dose to the patient.
E. Increasing the exposure time might result in increased patient dose.

28. The thermal rating of an x-ray tube used in diagnostic radiology:

A. Is limited by the maximum allowable filament current at high kV.
B. Is greater when operated at full-wave rectification compared to half-wave at an exposure of 0.1 sec.
C. Is influenced by anode angle.
D. Increases if the speed of rotation decreases.
E. Is, with respect to multiple exposures, dependent on the weight of the anode.

29. Regarding x-ray tube ratings:

A. Only thermal ratings are important.

B. During screening, the heat capacity of the tube housing limits the maximum tube current at a given kVp.

C. At very short exposures, three phase rectified x-ray tubes are rated higher than full-wave rectified tubes.

D. When multiple short exposures are taken, more heat may arise from the anode motor than from x-ray production.

E. A rotating anode has improved efficiency of heat production compared with a stationary anode.

30. The heat rating of an x-ray tube:

A. Decreases as the kV is increased.

B. Increases as exposure time is lengthened.

C. Is greater for a high speed anode.

D. Is greater for a stationary anode than for a rotating one.

E. Increases with an increase in effective focal spot size.

chapter 4

IMAGE QUALITY AND X-RAY PRODUCTION

ANSWERS

1. A. True: Compton reaction is proportionally higher for soft tissue at 40keV.
B. True: The approximate mean atomic number of bone is 13.8 and of soft tissue is 7.4.
C. True.
D. True.
E. False: MAC = LAC/density.

Allisy-Roberts & Williams. *Farr's Physics for Medical Imaging*, 2nd edn, Saunders Elsevier, 2008. pp. 9–10.

2. A. True: Beam quality = kVp + HVL.
B. True: Beam intensity is the energy fluence rate. It is the total amount of energy per unit area passing through a cross section per unit time. It depends on tube current, atomic number and is inversely proportional to the square of the distance from a point source.
C. False.
D. True.
E. True.

Electronic Learning Database, E-Learning for Healthcare, Radiology—Integrated Training Initiative (R-ITI) – www.e-lfh.org.uk
Module: 8a_065_Image Quality.

3. A. True: Assuming the x-ray beam is traversing a homogenous medium.
B. True: As electron density increases, more photons are attenuated.
C. False: Photoelectric interactions occur more for bone than soft tissue between 20 and 100keV.
D. False: The units of MAC are centimetres (squared)/kg.
E. True.

4. A. True: MAC= LAC/density.
B. True: MAC is not affected by density. It is affected only by atomic number and photon energy.
C. False: HVL = 0.69/LAC and since LAC is proportional to MAC then MAC is inversely proportional to HVL.
D. False: This is only the case for elastic scattering (all energies) and Compton interactions involving photons >100keV.
E. True.

Dendy, P. P. & Heaton, B. *Physics for Diagnostic Radiology*, 2nd edn, IOP Publishing Ltd., 1999. pp. 60–1.

5. A. True.
B. True.
C. True.
D. True.
E. True: As the angle of scatter of a photon increases, more energy is lost from the photon.

Learning Points

Attenuation coefficients and half value thickness

Linear attenuation coefficient (LAC) applies to narrow monoenergetic beams and measures the probability that a photon interacts per unit length of the path it travels in a specified material.

LAC increases as the density of the material increases, as atomic number increases and as photon energy of radiation decreases.

MAC stands for mass attenuation coefficient.

MAC = LAC / density

Most beloved MCQ question is the fact that MAC is independent of density and depends ***only*** on the atomic number and photon energy.

HVL stands for half value layer. This is the thickness of a known absorbing material required to reduce the incident radiation by half of the original. For a diagnostic energy range, HVL is measured in millimetres of aluminium.

HVL = 0.69/u (LAC)

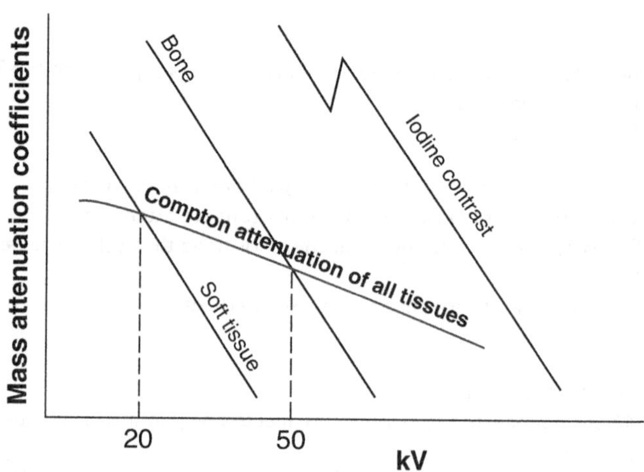

Figure 4.1 Photoelectric and Compton mass attenuation coefficients of materials of different atomic numbers at different photon energies
Allisy-Roberts & Williams. *Farr's Physics for Medical Imaging*, 2nd edn, Saunders Elsevier, 2008. p. 53.

6. A. False.
B. False.
C. True.
D. False.
E. False.

7. A. False: High kV increases scatter production.
B. True: A moving grid prevents some scatter and some primary radiation from reaching the film.
C. True.
D. False: This does not change the amount of scatter reaching the film.
E. True: All radiation is attenuated more therefore less scatter reaches the film as the zinc sheet is between the scatter and the film.

Electronic Learning Database, E-Learning for Healthcare, Radiology—Integrated Training Initiative (R-ITI) – www.e-lfh.org.uk
Module: 8a_065_Image Quality.
Allisy-Roberts & Williams. *Farr's Physics for Medical Imaging*, 2nd edn, Saunders Elsevier, 2008. pp. 54–6.

8. A. True.
B. True.
C. False.
D. True.
E. False: Grid lines can occur with a moving grid as it is momentarily stationary as it changes direction.

Allisy-Roberts & Williams. *Farr's Physics for Medical Imaging*, 2nd edn, Saunders Elsevier, 2008. p. 55.

9. A. True: Usual interspace materials are plastic, carbon fibre, or aluminium.
B. True.
C. True.
D. True.
E. False: A crossed grid is two stationary grids superimposed with their grid lines at right angles to each other. The radiation must pass though a tunnel rather than just a channel. Crossed grids require higher exposure and careful centring. If the grids are not at right angles an artefact called Moiré fringes may be visualized on the film.

Electronic Learning Database, E-Learning for Healthcare, Radiology—Integrated Training Initiative (R-ITI) – www.e-lfh.org.uk
Module: 8a_067: Intensifying Screens and Anti-Scatter Grids

10. A. False: The patient gets the same or more scatter due to the higher dose needed when using a grid.
B. False: This is inherent to the film screen.
C. True: More x-rays are needed to obtain the same film density when a grid sits between the film and the patient.
D. True: The beam becomes more penetrating as lower energy radiation cannot reach the film.
E. True.

Sherer, Visconti, and Ritenour. *Radiation Protection in Medical Radiography*, 4th edn, Mosby, 2002. pp. 174–5.

11. A. False.
B. True.
C. True.
D. False.
E. True.

Electronic Learning Database, E-Learning for Healthcare, Radiology—Integrated Training Initiative (R-ITI) – www.e-lfh.org.uk
Module: 8a_067: Intensifying Screens and Anti-Scatter Grids.

12. A. True: This removes low energy photons which contribute to dose but not to the image.
B. True: This is a tricky question. It requires you to understand that kVp and mAs are intrinsically linked. It is usually assumed that when the kVp is increased that the mAs is reduced and vice versa. This will often not be stated in the question. So as kVp increases, mAs concomitantly decreases.
C. False: This increases dose to the patient.
D. True: Rare earth screens are more efficient that calcium tungstate, therefore less x-rays are needed for the same image. The downside of this is that noise is increased as fewer photons contribute to the image.
E. False: A Potter-Bucky grid is the term used to describe the moving grid assembly.

Allisy-Roberts & Williams. *Farr's Physics for Medical Imaging*, 2nd edn, Saunders Elsevier, 2008. pp. 66–7.

13. A. True.
B. True: As grid height increases, more scattered radiation is stopped and resolution improves. However, primary radiation is also stopped and so a higher dose is incurred.
C. False: Grid factor is the ratio of exposure needed with a grid/exposure needed without a grid. The usual ratio is 2–6.
D. True.
E. False: This is primary transmission.

Dendy, P. P. & Heaton, B. *Physics for Diagnostic Radiology*, 2nd edn, IOP Publishing Ltd., 1999. pp. 122–5.

14. A. True: The penumbra is a consequence of the focal spot. The penumbra is the zone of unsharpness that represents the area at which the margins caused by many point sources of x-rays in the focal spot overlap.
B. True: Any motion of the x-ray tube components or patient contributes to motion unsharpness.
C. False: Absorption unsharpness is caused by attenuation around the object being imaged – not the focal spot.
D. False: Due to the anode heel effect, the intensity of radiation varies across the face of the focal spot.
E. True.

Allisy-Roberts & Williams. *Farr's Physics for Medical Imaging*, 2nd edn, Saunders Elsevier, 2008. pp. 57–8.

15. A. True: Blooming (an increase in focal spot size) occurs when there is an increase in mA or a low kV, especially noticeable with small focal spots.
B. False: Resolution is measured with a star test pattern. Focal spot size is measured with pinhole imaging.
C. False: This has no impact on the focal spot size.
D. False.
E. True.

Learning Points

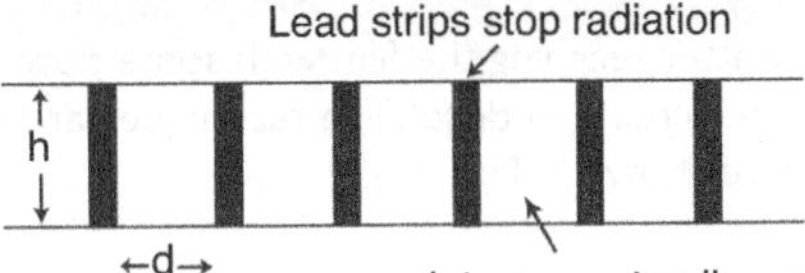

Grids are not used in paediatric patients due to the increased dose needed. The increase in dose can be up to four times compared to without a grid.

Parallel grid:
There is a reduction of optical density towards the film edges.

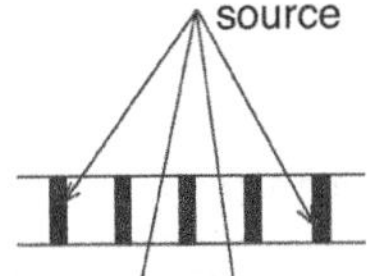

Focused grid:
There are parallel to the x-rays across the film but only within a narrow range of focus to film distances.

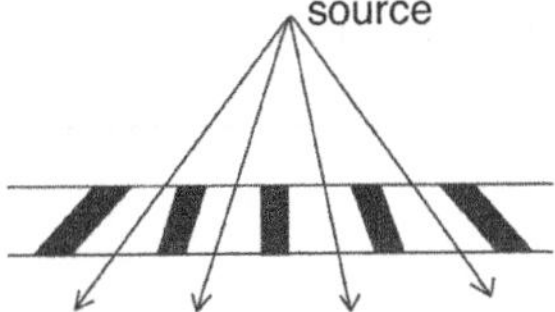

GRID RATIO = h/d

$$\textbf{Grid Factor} = \frac{\textbf{Exposure needed with a grid}}{\textbf{Exposure needed without a grid}}$$

Figure 4.2 Grids

Dendy, P. P. & Heaton, B. *Physics for Diagnostic Radiology*, 2nd edn, IOP Publishing Ltd., 1999. pp. 52–5.
Sherer, Visconti, and Ritenour. *Radiation Protection in Medical Radiography*, 4th edn, Mosby, 2002. pp. 174–5.

Focal Spot

A small focal spot means a sharp image.

As focal spot size increases:

- local heating of the x-ray tube decreases;
- geometric unsharpness increases.

Focal spot is measured by:

- Pinhole camera – for actual focal spot size;
- Star test object – to measure the resolving capacity of the focal spot.

Blooming refers to the increase in focal spot size which occurs when the tube is operated at high mA. It occurs more at low kV with small focal spots.

Dendy, P. P. & Heaton, B. *Physics for Diagnostic Radiology*, 2nd edn, IOP Publishing Ltd., 1999. pp. 52–5.

Learning Points *(continued)*

Air gap

This technique can reduce scatter reaching the film with some dose saving (compared to using a grid which requires an increase in dose). The technique can be recalled in the exam by reproducing the simple picture shown in Figure 4.3.

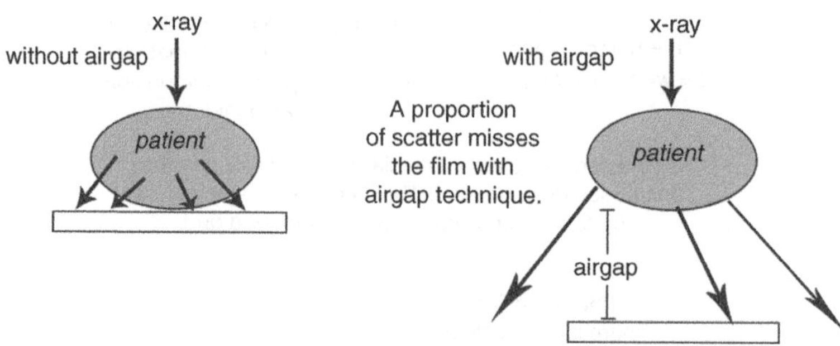

Figure 4.3 The effect of air gap

Allisy-Roberts & Williams. *Farr's Physics for Medical Imaging*, 2nd edn, Saunders Elsevier, 2008. pp. 55.
Sherer, Visconti, and Ritenour. *Radiation Protection in Medical Radiography*, 4th edn, Mosby, 2002. pp. 175–6.

16. A. True.
B. False.
C. True.
D. True.
E. True.

17. A. False: Scatter is not *removed.* The scatter that misses the film does not contribute to the image but scatter which does not lie obliquely contributes to the image.
B. True: With a gap of less than 30cm, too much scatter reaches the film to be a valued technique.
C. False: Grids require a higher patient dose than air gap.
D. False: Grids are not used on paediatric patients due to the need for a higher exposure.
E. True.

Sherer, Visconti, and Ritenour. *Radiation Protection in Medical Radiography*, 4th edn, Mosby, 2002. pp. 175–6.

18. A. True: The x-ray tube and the cassette move in a fixed arc in *opposite* directions relative to each other, but centred around the object of interest.
B. False: A large swing angle produces a thinner slice.
C. True: Peripherally, tissues are blurred with the object of interest in focus. However this reduces contrast.
D. True.
E. True.

Allisy-Roberts & Williams. *Farr's Physics for Medical Imaging*, 2nd edn, Saunders Elsevier, 2008. pp. 76–7.

19. A. True.
B. False: Structures at right angles appear more blurred than those parallel to the film.
C. False: It is most useful when imaging structures with high inherent contrast.
D. False.
E. True.

20. A. True.
B. False: Tissue contrast is enhanced. Narrow angle tomography is preferred when imaging tissue of low inherent contrast.
C. False: Decreased.
D. False: Decreased.
E. True: This can be compensated for by using multidirectional tomography.

Electronic Learning Database, E-Learning for Healthcare, Radiology—Integrated Training Initiative (R-ITI) – www.e-lfh.org.uk
Module 8a_074: Tomography.

21. A. False: Rotating the anode makes no difference to the size of the focal spot.
B. True: Heat is spread over the track of the rotating anode. It can withstand much larger exposures without focal spot damage.
C. True: A stationary anode allows only slow heat removal by conduction, restricting the maximum exposures that can be made. Stationary anode tubes are only used now for intra-oral dental sets and some mobile units.
D. False.
E. False: The anode can be made from rhodium and the target from both molybedenum or rhodium in mammography.

Allisy-Roberts & Williams. *Farr's Physics for Medical Imaging*, 2nd edn, Saunders Elsevier, 2008. pp. 59–60.

22. A. False: It is made of molybdenum which is a poor thermal conductor.
B. True.
C. False: Heat is lost mainly by radiation. It cannot be removed by convection as the rotating anode lies within a vacuum.
D. False: If a high current is used, heat is removed more efficiently.
E. True.

Allisy-Roberts & Williams. *Farr's Physics for Medical Imaging*, 2nd edn, Saunders Elsevier, 2008. pp. 59–60.

23. A. False: Inherent filtration is the absorption of x-rays within the x-ray tube.
B. False: Filtration increases the mean energy of the beam therefore decreasing tissue contrast.
C. False: Aluminium atomic no is 13 and copper is 29 so copper attenuates x-rays more by photoelectric effect.
D. False: Maximum photon energy stays the same – filtration preferentially filters lower energy photons that results in a higher mean energy.
E. False: Filtration increases the loading on the tube because it increases the mean photon energy, so giving higher output intensity.

Dendy, P. P. & Heaton, B. *Physics for Diagnostic Radiology*, 2nd edn, IOP Publishing Ltd., 1999. pp. 75–8.

Learning Points

Which angle are they talking about when they ask questions about the anode angle?

This is important and it is easy to get mixed up, thinking of the wrong angle.

Definitions

Actual focal spot: the actual area of the focal spot on the radiographic target as viewed at right angles to the plane of the target.

Effective focal spot: The face of the anode that carries the target in an x-ray tube is slanted from the vertical to increase the volume of the target but to reduce the size of the origin of the x-ray beam (Figure 4.4).

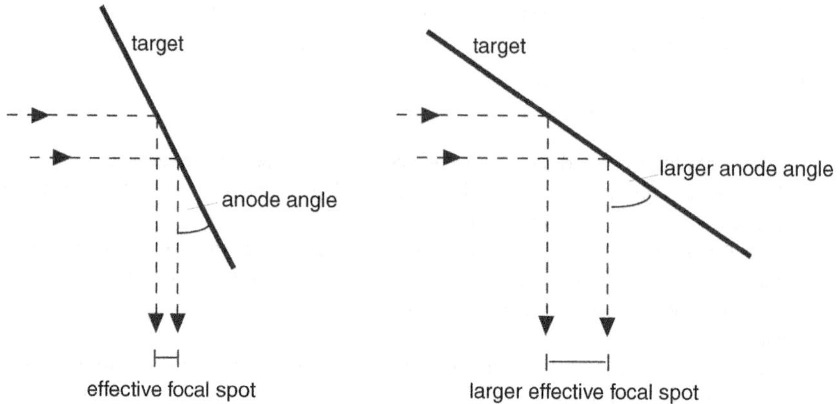

Figure 4.4 Anode angle

As the anode angle increases, the effective focal spot increases in size (the actual focal spot remains the same).

The anode angle will normally vary between 6 and 15 degrees.

Allisy-Roberts & Williams. *Farr's Physics for Medical Imaging*, 2nd edn, Saunders Elsevier, 2008. pp. 58–9.

24. A. True: Inherent filtration is the combined filtration of the window of the tube housing, the insulating oil, the glass insert and the target material itself.
B. True.
C. True.
D. True: Beryllium has an atomic number of 4 and is used where inherent filtration must be minimized, e.g. in mammography.
E. True.

Electronic Learning Database, E-Learning for Healthcare, Radiology—Integrated Training Initiative (R-ITI) – www.e-lfh.org.uk
Module 8a_069: Factors Affecting Image Quality.

25. A. True: In fluoroscopy the effective focal spot is usually 0.6mm (actual focal spot can vary up to 50% from manufacturers' specifications).
B. True: This is where the beam is most useful.
C. True: Rotating anodes increase the area over which heat is produced so helping to dissipate heat.
D. True: Rhenium is added to prevent cracking of the anode.
E. False.

26. A. True.
B. False.
C. False.
D. False.
E. False.

27. A. True: As mAs decreases.
B. True: As mAs must decrease to achieve the same film density.
C. True.
D. True.
E. True.

28. A. False.
B. False.
C. True.
D. False.
E. True.

29. A. False: Electrical ratings are important too.
B. False: The anode heat storage capacity is the limiting factor. The tube housing heat capacity is much higher.
C. True.
D. True.
E. False: Regardless of the type of anode, the efficiency of heat production is largely similar – with over 99% of energy lost as heat.

30. A. True: As kV increases, mAs is decreased. The higher the mAs used, the more effective heat removal is.
B. False.
C. True.
D. False.
E. True.

Electronic Learning Database, E-Learning for Healthcare, Radiology—Integrated Training Initiative (R-ITI) – www.e-lfh.org.uk
Module: 8a_063: Heat Removal (Thermal Loading).
Allisy-Roberts & Williams. *Farr's Physics for Medical Imaging*, 2nd edn, Saunders Elsevier, 2008. pp. 60–1.

chapter 5

FILM SCREEN RADIOGRAPHY

QUESTIONS

1. Regarding intensifying screens:

A. Calcium tungstate emits blue light.
B. The light production efficiency of a calcium tungstate intensifying screen is 5%.
C. They emit electrons when bombarded with x-rays.
D. The intensification factor is not related to patient dose.
E. Shorter exposures can be used.

2. Photographic density:

A. Is measured objectively only.
B. Is a measure of the blackness of a film.
C. The useful density range on a diagnostic x-ray film is between 0.25–2.
D. The film base contributes a density of about 0.07.
E. Film fog on an unexposed film contributes a density of about 0.05.

3. Base plus fog is:

A. Affected by developer temperature.
B. Affected by moving grids.
C. The optical density of the base, plus the exposed film emulsion.
D. Influenced by background radiation.
E. Increased by storage in damp conditions.

4. If x-ray film is replaced by one with greater latitude:

A. The range of optical densities in the image will be greater.
B. The contrast in the image will be increased.
C. Errors in setting the exposure (mAs) are less likely to produce an incorrectly exposed film.
D. A larger exposure (mAs) is needed to give an exposure of correct density.
E. It is less likely that an anti-scatter grid will be needed.

5. In the construction of x-ray film:

A. Cellulose triacetate is the main material currently used for film bases.
B. The emulsion layer normally consists of silver halide crystals suspended in gelatine.
C. Intra-oral dental films are usually single emulsion films.
D. Panchromatic emulsions must be handled in complete darkness.
E. 105mm roll film used in spot film cameras has a width of 105mm.

6. In films used in radiography:

A. The emulsion crystals contain more iodide than bromide.
B. The latent image is produced at the sensitivity specks.
C. The screen coating the posterior emulsion functions by absorbing light produced by the anterior emulsion.
D. The agent in the development process that produces the silver metallic grains from the latent image should be an electron donor.
E. Increasing the developer temperature would be expected to increase the speed of the film.

7. Regarding the structure of the film:

A. Polyester would be a suitable material for the film base.
B. Silver iodide halides in the crystals function as sensitivity specks.
C. Each grain consists of about 1000 neutral atoms.
D. The probability of development of a latent image centre is independent of the number of silver atoms present at the latent image centre.
E. A single absorbed x-ray photon will result in the migration of more silver atoms than a single absorbed light photon.

8. Regarding the properties of film:

A. A narrow grain distribution results in higher contrast characteristics.
B. The sensitivity of the emulsion is independent of grain size.
C. The use of duplicated film results in a reduced patient dose.
D. Non-screen films have a role in oral dental radiography.
E. The optical density of the image may be measured with a sensitometer.

9. When x-rays are generated at 50kV using a tungsten target and aluminium filter:

A. The maximum photon energy will be 50keV.
B. The spectrum will have its maximum intensity at 50keV.
C. Characteristic radiation from the tube is not present in the radiation emitted from the tube.
D. X-ray output (dose per mAs) will be decreased if the filter thickness is increased.
E. The K-edge of the filter is important in shaping the x-ray spectrum.

10. The characteristic curve of the film screen system:

A. Is derived by exposing the system to a series of exposures.
B. Is the plot of a log of the optical density against the log relative exposure.
C. The base density is greater in tinted films.
D. The average gradient of the curve is independent of the grain size.
E. The curve moves to the right as sensitivity increases.

11. Fog level:

A. Exposure fog decreases radiographic contrast.
B. True fog is increased by exhausted developer.
C. High speed films are less likely to be fogged by excessive development temperature than slower films.
D. Fog may change the gamma of a film.
E. Fog mostly affects the contrast between high densities.

12. Subject contrast is generally decreased by:

A. Film fog.
B. Tissues with similar densities.
C. Using 30kVp instead of 60kVp in mammography.
D. Use of contrast media.
E. Using a lower total exposure (mAs).

13. Radiographic contrast would increase if:

A. kV is increased.
B. Compression is applied.
C. A grid is used.
D. Field size is limited.
E. mAs is decreased.

14. In film screen radiography, image unsharpness may be affected by:

A. The adequacy of film screen contact.
B. Geometric magnification.
C. Focal spot size.
D. Grain size in the emulsion.
E. The use of tomography.

15. The following factors would be expected to lead to a loss of sharpness in a film screen system:

A. A shorter exposure time.
B. A larger focal spot.
C. Increased magnification.
D. Imaging round rather than square images.
E. Using a double emulsion film instead of a single emulsion film.

16. Geometrical unsharpness is influenced by:

A. Focus–film distance.
B. Focal spot size.
C. The type of screen used.
D. The thickness of the patient.
E. The object–film distance.

17. Unsharpness:

A. Unsharpness will be masked by low contrast.
B. Geometric unsharpness is reduced by keeping magnification as low as possible.
C. Motion unsharpness may be caused by tube movement.
D. Absorption sharpness is greatest when sharp edges in the subject are exposed.
E. Parallax unsharpness may be seen in single emulsion films.

18. Radiographic mottle in an x-ray image:

A. In film screen radiography, is affected by sensitivity variations in the intensifying screen.
B. Limits resolution in low contrast images.
C. In film screen radiography, can be reduced by employing a screen with a greater (x-ray to light) conversion factor.
D. Structural mottle is more significant than radiographic mottle in a radiographic image.
E. Radiographic mottle is made worse using a fast film screen combination.

19. Radiographic mottle in a radiographic image will be increased by (assume that exposure factors are adjusted to keep the film density constant, except in 'E'):

A. Using a screen with a higher conversion efficiency.
B. Using a thicker screen.
C. Using a higher speed film.
D. Increasing the focus film distance.
E. In computed radiography, increasing the exposure (mAs).

20. Radiographic mottle (noise) in an intensifying screen:

A. Contributes significantly to the total screen mottle.
B. Is caused mainly by variations in the thickness of the phosphor layer.
C. Is most likely to compromise images with higher contrast.
D. Is increased by using a phosphor with a higher x-ray to light conversion efficiency.
E. Is increased by using a phosphor with increased thickness.

21. In macro radiography:

A. The tube effective focal spot should be less than one centimetre.
B. The film–patient distance should be as small as possible.
C. The mA should be relatively small.
D. The resolution of the final image is generally limited by grain size.
E. Magnification reduces the modulation transfer function (MTF) of the screen.

22. Regarding modulation transfer function of a screen-film system:

A. It usually ranges from 0.1 to 2.
B. It may be calculated from the line spread function of the system.
C. It may be calculated from the Wiener spectrum of the system.
D. It is defined as the representation of the system's ability to resolve 1 line pair per mm at different kVp values.
E. It is equal to the exposure amplitude output over the exposure amplitude input.

23. Regarding production of an x-ray image:

A. Low kV techniques increase the amount of forward scatter.
B. In radiography of the hand, use of a grid is highly recommended.
C. In macro radiography an air gap is used primarily to decrease the amount of scatter.
D. Geometric unsharpness depends on the tube target angle.
E. The resolution limit of a system is equal to the spatial frequency that corresponds to an MTF of 1.

24. Advantages of high kV radiography include:

A. Scattered radiation is increased.
B. Reducing the differential absorption of soft tissue to bone.
C. Radiation dose to the patient is reduced.
D. Greater exposure latitude.
E. Reducing the electrical loading of the x-ray tube.

25. High kV technique:

A. Gives wider exposure latitude.
B. Air-gap technique is used.
C. Heat loading of the x-ray tube is increased.
D. Gives a higher skin dose.
E. Increases scatter production.

26. Comparing x-ray mammography with conventional film screen radiography:

A. X-rays with a lower mean photon energy are used.
B. Shorter exposure times are used.
C. A larger focal spot is used.
D. A shorter focus-film distance is used.
E. An anti-scatter grid is less likely to be used.

27. In a mammographic x-ray set with a molybdenum target:

A. The x-ray spectrum is generally dominated by characteristic radiation.
B. The typical tube potential for mammographic exposures is about 35kV.
C. The anode does not rotate.
D. The radiation detector for the automatic exposure control is between the grid and the cassette.
E. The filter may also be molybdenum.

28. When compression is used in mammography:

A. It reduces the dose to the breast.
B. Its prime purpose is to immobilize the patient.
C. It reduces the proportion of scattered radiation reaching the film screen.
D. It reduced the total volume of the breast.
E. The applied force must be less than 50N (5kg force).

29. Mammography:

A. Maximum image contrast is obtained at photon energies of 50–60keV.
B. The characteristic radiation of a molybdenum target occurs at 17.5 and 19.5keV.
C. The molybdenum filter attenuates the characteristic radiation produced by a molybdenum target.
D. General mammography uses a focal spot of 1mm.
E. The average dose per mammogram to glandular breast tissue is 2mGy.

30. In xeroradiography:

A. Double emulsion film is used.
B. The final image is transferred to paper.
C. Wet processing is required for development of the image.
D. Gives a lower dose than in film screen radiography.
E. The edges of a structure are enhanced.

chapter

5

FILM SCREEN RADIOGRAPHY

ANSWERS

1. A. True.
B. True: Light production efficiency of a calcium tungstate screen is only 5%, while rare earth screens are better at 20%.
C. True: Intensifying screens are fluorescent and emit light when x-rays strike. However, they also emit electrons because x-rays undergo Compton scatter and photoelectric absorption in detector materials.
D. False: As intensification factor increases, the dose needed to produce an adequate image reduces.
E. True: Thus minimizing movement unsharpness.

Electronic Learning Database, E-Learning for Healthcare, Radiology—Integrated Training Initiative (R-ITI) – www.e-lfh.org.uk
Module: 8a_067 Intensifying Screens and Anti-Scatter Grids.

2. A. False: This can be subjective and objective – measured by eye or by densimetry.
B. True.
C. True: The useful density range is 0.25–2; <0.25 too light; >2 too dark.
D. True.
E. True.

3. A. True.
B. False: Moving grids reduce contrast in the final image but do not affect the base plus fog level.
C. False: It is the optical density of the base plus the unexposed film.
D. True: High amounts of background radiation increases fog.
E. True.

Allisy-Roberts & Williams. *Farr's Physics for Medical Imaging*, 2nd edn, Saunders Elsevier, 2008. pp. 68–9.

4. A. False: The range remains the same.
B. False: The contrast would be decreased.
C. True: The wider range of exposures in the latitude means that a high or low mAs may still lie within the latitude and produce a change in optical density.
D. False.
E. False.

Sherer, Visconti, and Ritenour. *Radiation Protection in Medical Radiography*, 4th edn, Mosby, 2002. pp. 173–4.

5. A. False: Polyester has replaced cellulose triacetate as the base – chosen for its strength and stability.
B. True.
C. False: Dental films use double emulsion but do not use intensifying screens.
D. True: Making them less popular as a film choice despite their superior sensitivity.
E. True.

Electronic Learning Database, E-Learning for Healthcare, Radiology—Integrated Training Initiative (R-ITI) – www.e-lfh.org.uk
Module: 8a_064: X-Ray Film.

Learning Points

Intensifying screens

Intensifying screens convert x-rays to light and manage to convert 1 photon to about 1500 light photons. They can absorb 20–40 times more x-rays than film. They allow a smaller exposure for the same image density. They are the largest contribution to reduction in dose. Common screen materials are:

Calcium tungstate	Z = 74	emits blue light
Gadolinium oxysulphate with terbium	Z = 64	emits green light
Lanthanum oxysulphide	Z = 57	emits blue light

Rare earth – despite the name these are not actually that rare and are in the earth in abundance.

Advantages of intensifying screens

- Lower patient dose;
- Shorter exposure time and therefore less motion artefact;
- Better image contrast.

Disadvantages of intensifying screens

- Poorer spatial resolution;
- Noise is increased as fewer photons contribute to the image.

Intensification factor

This is a measure of the speed of a pair of screens. It measures the reduction in patient dose and tube loading when screens are used:

$$\frac{\text{air kerma to produce D = 1 with film alone}}{\text{air kerma to produce D = 1 with film and screens}}$$

Intensification factor increases when:

- kV increases;
- Phosphor thickness increases;
- Crystal size increases;
- When a white reflecting layer between the base and the phosphor is used;
- When a rare earth screen is used instead of calcium tungstate.

6. A. False: The emulsion contains 90% silver bromide and 10% silver iodide.
B. True: Electrons liberated by light photons migrate to the sensitivity speck and attract mobile silver with them. The silver ions accumulated at this speck form the latent image used to form the final image in development.
C. False.
D. True: The agent in development needs to be an electron donor to reduce the positive silver ions to silver metal grains.
E. True: Increasing developer temperature increases the rate of chemical reaction and so increases the film speed.

Electronic Learning Database, E-Learning for Healthcare, Radiology—Integrated Training Initiative (R-ITI) – www.e-lfh.org.uk
Module: 8a_064: X-Ray Film.

7. A. True: Polyester is most commonly used for its strength and stability.
B. False: Sensitivity specks are due to crystal structure imperfection.
C. False: Each grain has silver ions.
D. False: The probability of latent image development is dependent on the number of silver atoms present.
E. True.

Sherer, Visconti, and Ritenour. *Radiation Protection in Medical Radiography*, 4th edn, Mosby, 2002. pp. 173–4.

8. A. True: All grains change within a narrow range of photon energies.
B. False: Sensitivity is dependent on grain size.
C. True: As optical densities are additive, duplicated film results in a lower dose for the same density film.
D. True: Intra-oral dental radiography uses double emulsion but no screens.
E. False: Measured with a densitometer.

Electronic Learning Database, E-Learning for Healthcare, Radiology—Integrated Training Initiative (R-ITI) – www.e-lfh.org.uk
Module 8a_064: X-ray Film.

9. A. True: The given kV for a tube describes its maximum photon energy. The maximum photon energy cannot be above this. However the mean energy of the photon will be much lower. Hence B is false.
B. False: Remembering the characteristic x-ray spectrum, the mean photon energy is usually about a third of its maximum energy.
C. True: Characteristic radiation only occurs when the photon energy is high enough.
D. True: If filter thickness increases, more low energy photons are removed from the beam, therefore the area under the curve decreases.
E. False: Not in this instance, as at 50kV the energy is not high enough to produce tungsten characteristic radiation that occurs at 70kV or above.

10. A. True.
B. False: The graph is *optical density* against log relative exposure.
C. True: The tinted polyester base increases absorption.
D. False: Grain size is an important factor in determining gradient.
E. False: The curve becomes less sensitive as it moves to the right.

Dendy, P. P. & Heaton, B. *Physics for Diagnostic Radiology*, 2nd edn, IOP Publishing Ltd., 1999. pp. 89–93.

Learning Points

X-ray film

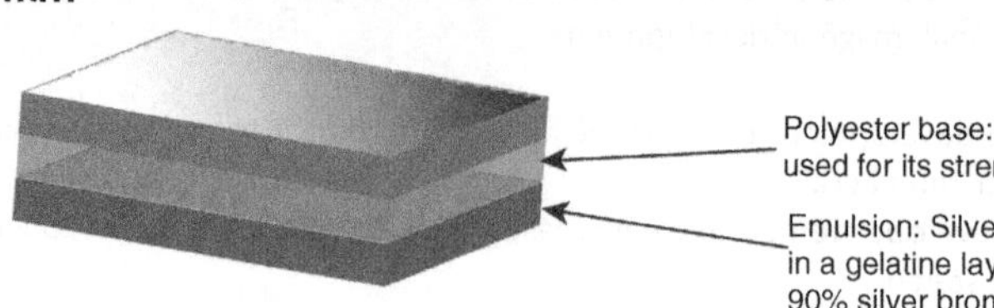
Polyester base: 150 micrometer thick, used for its strength and stability
Emulsion: Silver halide with impurities in a gelatine layer.
90% silver bromide, 10% silver iodide

Figure 5.1 X-ray plate

Grain development

- Unexposed:
  - Silver bromide grain at microscopic level,
  - Free Ag+ and Br–,
  - Sensitive spot is due to crystal structure imperfection;
- Exposure:
  - Light absorbed by Br,
  - Electrons are free and get trapped by sensitive spot,
  - Silver ions attract to spot and are neutralized,
  - Atom of black metallic silver formed;
- Repeated exposure:
  - Process repeated,
  - Metallic silver atoms form a latent image,
  - 10–80 atoms make the grain developable;
- Development:
  - Developer solution supplies electrons,
  - Electrons migrate to the sensitive spot,
  - Silver ions are now converted to black metallic silver and a visible image is seen.

Learning Points *(continued)*

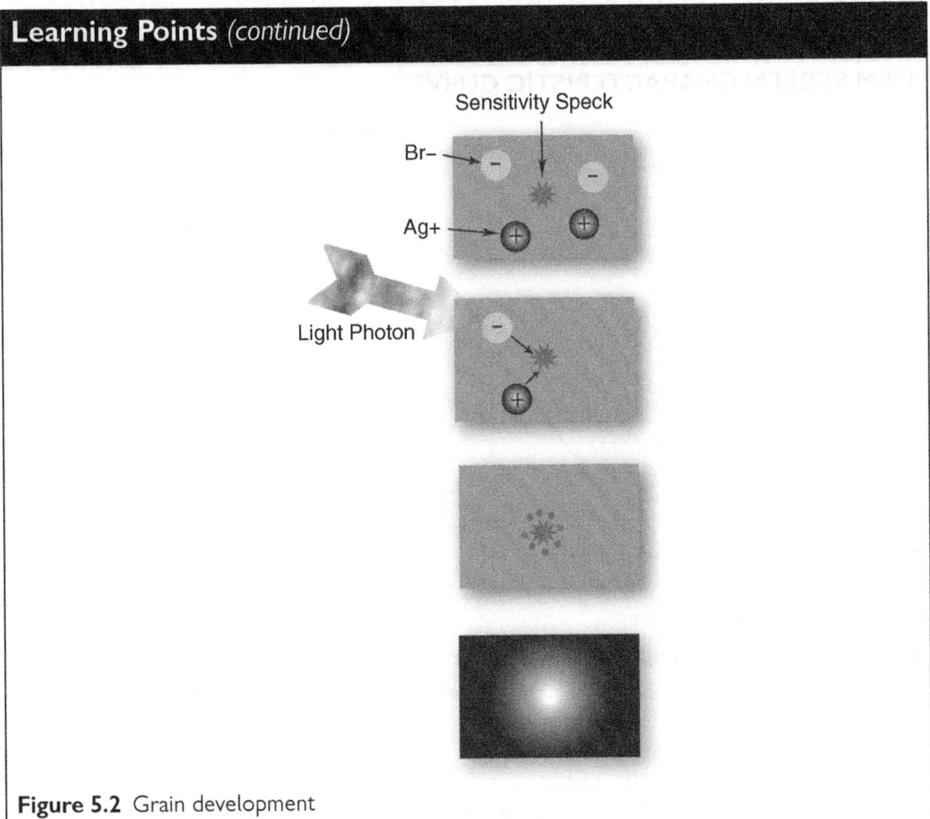

Figure 5.2 Grain development

Learning Points

FILM SCREEN CHARACTERISTIC CURVE

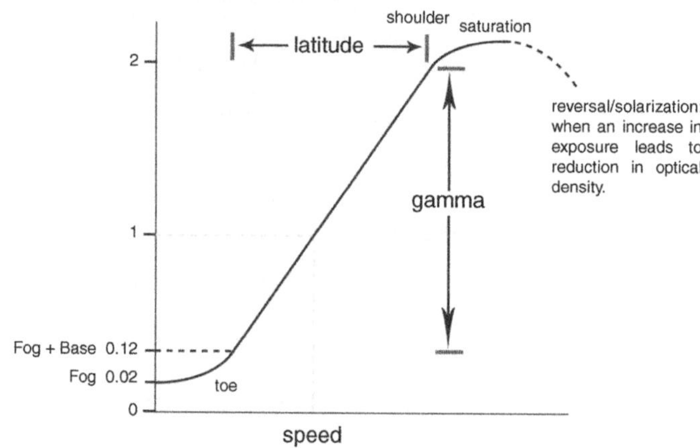

Figure 5.3 Absorption/edge unsharpness

Table 5.1 Definition of terms

Fog level	Density of processed but unexposed film – inherent fog 0.12.
Speed	Reciprocal of air kerma needed to produce D = 1 (average density of the exposed film) affected by: •Photon energy •Thicker/presence of screen •Atomic no of screen material •Film grain shape •Concentration/time/temperature of developer
Gamma	Slope of straight line portion 0.2–2.
Film latitude	Or dynamic range – this is the range of exposures lying in the useful density range 0.25–2. As film latitude increases, gamma decreases.
Exposure latitude	The range of exposure factors (kV, mAs) which will give correct exposure of a given subject. This depends on film screen latitude and gamma and on subject contrast.
Optical density	This is a measure of the blackening of an area of film. Darkness of the film increases as exposure increases. D = log10 (incident light/transmitted light) It depends on the number of silver grains per unit area and is measured by a densitometer.

11. A. True.
B. True.
C. False: High speed films are likely to be more sensitive.
D. False: Gamma is the gradient, the addition of extra fog will not change it.
E. False: It mostly affects the contrast between low densities.

Allisy-Roberts & Williams. *Farr's Physics for Medical Imaging*, 2nd edn, Saunders Elsevier, 2008. pp. 68–73.

12. A. False: Film fog influences final *radiographic* contrast but does not influence *subject* contrast.
B. True.
C. True.
D. False: This increases subject contrast by increasing photoelectric effect.
E. False: Total exposure affects film density but does not affect the subject contrast.

Allisy-Roberts & Williams. *Farr's Physics for Medical Imaging*, 2nd edn, Saunders Elsevier, 2008. pp. 70–1.

13. A. False: Scatter increases with increased kV therefore reducing contrast.
B. True: Thinner section of tissue is imaged so less scatter is produced giving improved contrast.
C. True: Reduces scatter reaching the film.
D. True: Reduced field size therefore reduces scatter.
E. False: As mAs decreases, radiographic contrast reduces.

Dendy, P. P. & Heaton, B. *Physics for Diagnostic Radiology*, 2nd edn, IOP Publishing Ltd., 1999. pp. 116–17.

14. A. True: Poor contact increases unsharpness. Film screen contact is tested with a wire mesh.
B. True.
C. True: Affects geometrical unsharpness.
D. True: As grain size increases, unsharpness increases and resolution is poorer but sensitivity improves.
E. True: By its nature give blurring around the object being imaged. Contrast is also reduced.

15. A. False: This reduces motion unsharpness.
B. True: This increases geometric unsharpness.
C. True: This increases geometric unsharpness.
D. True: This increases absorption unsharpness.
E. False: Using a double emulsion film causes a degree of parallax unsharpness, but this is usually negligible.

16. A. True.
B. True: This changes the penumbra.
C. False: No change.
D. False: Affects contrast but not unsharpness.
E. True.

17. A. True: Unsharpness is more noticeable when there is high contrast.
B. True.
C. True: Any movement of the patient or the tube or the film causes motion unsharpness.
D. False.
E. False: This occurs only in double emulsion films.

Electronic Learning Database, E-Learning for Healthcare, Radiology—Integrated Training Initiative (R-ITI) – www.e-lfh.org.uk
Module: 8a_069: Factors Affecting Image Quality.

Learning Points

CONTRAST

There are also different types of contrast and this point needs to be appreciated in order not to get caught out answering questions.

Table 5.2 Definitions of contrast

Subject contrast	Contrast inherent in the patient. Depends on • Thickness of structure • Difference in linear attenuation coefficients of tissues
Inherent contrast	This applies to the filtration of the absorbing of x-rays as they pass through the x-ray tube
Radiographic contrast	= radiation contrast × film contrast

UNSHARPNESS

There are different types of unsharpness, which are influenced by different factors. Questions tend to test whether this is understood.

Table 5.3 Types of unsharpness

Film screen	Loss of resolution due to screens. Light spreads out within the screen before reaching the film. Reduced by: • Thinner screen • Good film screen contact
Geometrical	This refers to the penumbra and is reduced by: • Smaller focal spot • Reduced object–film distance • Longer FFD
Movement	Movement is reduced by: • Immobilization • Shorter exposure time
Absorption/Patient	This refers to the gradual change in absorption near the edge of a tapered or rounded structure.
Parallax	Occurs in double emulsion systems. The rear emulsion film is slightly larger due to the divergence of the x-ray beam. This makes a small contribution, especially if the film is viewed obliquely.
Crossover	Occurs in double sided film where light from the upper intensifying screen sensitizes the lower screen and vice versa.

To minimize total unsharpness, the values of separate unsharpness components should approximate each other.

Learning Points

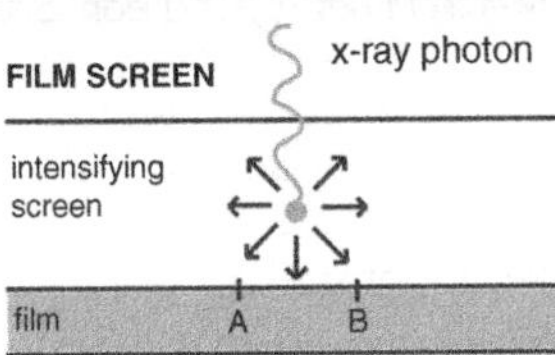

Light photons spread in all directions in the intensifying screen and strike anywhere in the film from A to B.

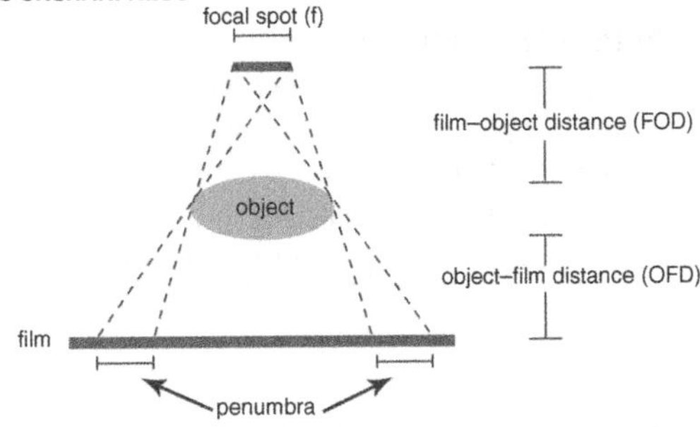

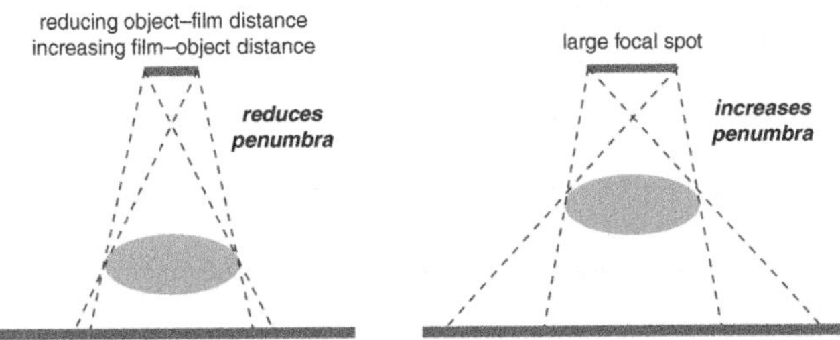

Diagrams are very helpful in these questions. Drawing a diagram like these an help you understand whether geometrical unsharpness is increased or decreased when focal spot size, focus film distance or an air gap is used. The relationships between these factors are summarized in the equation given.

$$\text{penumbra} \propto \frac{\text{focal spot . OFD}}{\text{FFD . FOD}}$$

Figure 5.4 Unsharpness

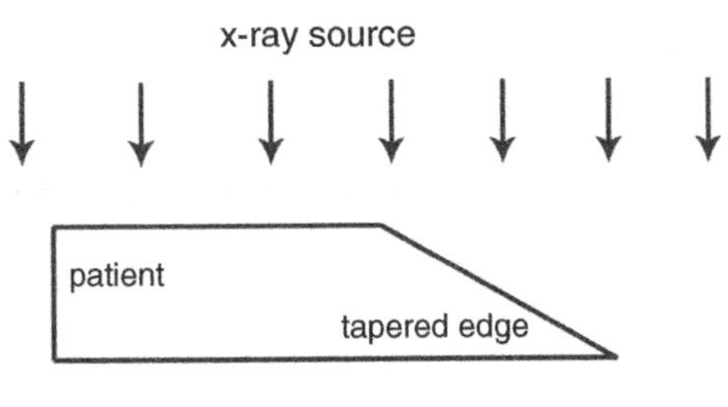

If an object has a tapering edge, the attenuation of x-ray gradually decreases towards the edge. This will produce a gradual change in optical density as shown.

Figure 5.5 Absorption/edge unsharpness

Learning Points *(continued)*

Allisy-Roberts & Williams. *Farr's Physics for Medical Imaging*, 2nd edn, Saunders Elsevier, 2008. pp. 57–58.

FOCAL SPOT SIZE

Focal spot size is measured by:

- Pinhole camera (which measures actual focal spot size).
- Star test object (which measures the resolving capacity of the focal spot).

Blooming refers to the increase in focal spot size which occurs when the tube is operated at high mA. It occurs more at low kV and with small focal spots.

QUANTUM MOTTLE/NOISE

This occurs due to the stochastic (random) nature of the x-ray attenuation process. A random pattern of photons is superimposed on the signal. This random pattern becomes more noticeable with low contrast structures.

(Structural mottle is another type, which occurs due to the fact that the screen is made up of individual crystals. This is not as important to the image as quantum mottle.)

18. A. False.
B. True.
C. False: Mottle or noise increases when a screen has a greater conversion factor. This produces an image with fewer photons.
D. False: Structural mottle is negligible compared with radiographic mottle.
E. True.

Allisy-Roberts & Williams. *Farr's Physics for Medical Imaging*, 2nd edn, Saunders Elsevier, 2008. p. 72.

19. A. True: Less photons are needed for the image so noise is more noticeable.
B. False.
C. True: Shorter exposure therefore less photons contribute to the image, thus increasing noise.
D. False: No change.
E. False: *In MCQ questions it is assumed that when mAs changes then so too does the kV, but in the opposite direction.* Thus increasing mAs means kV will decrease and there will be little change in the number of photons contributing to the image.

20. A. True: Radiographic mottle makes a larger contribution than structural mottle.
B. False: Variations in the thickness of the phosphor layer causes structural mottle.
C. False: Radiographic mottle is more noticeable at low contrast. At high contrast it is sharpness that limits the image.
D. True: Using a screen with better efficiency means that fewer photons are needed to produces an image so noise is increased.
E. False: Increasing screen thickness does not change noise but it will affect the sharpness of the image.

Allisy-Roberts & Williams. *Farr's Physics for Medical Imaging*, 2nd edn, Saunders Elsevier, 2008. pp. 72–3.

21. A. True.
B. False.
C. False.
D. False.
E. False: MTF is improved as the image is more representative of the actual object.

22. A. False.
B. True.
C. False.
D. False.
E. True.

Allisy-Roberts & Williams. *Farr's Physics for Medical Imaging*, 2nd edn, Saunders Elsevier, 2008. p. 83.

23. A. False: As kV increases, scatter increases and the proportion of that scatter that is forward is increased.
B. False: Grids are not used in paediatrics or on extremities.
C. False.
D. True.
E. False.

Dendy, P. P. & Heaton, B. *Physics for Diagnostic Radiology*, 2nd edn, IOP Publishing Ltd., 1999. pp. 241–3.

Learning Points

Modulation transfer function

This is often difficult to understand from conventional textbooks but is essentially really quite simple and is:

$$\frac{\text{Information in the image}}{\text{Information in the object imaged}}$$

It is a measure of how well a system reproduces the object it is imaging. It has no units and is a continuous function.

MTF of system = product of the MTFs of individual components

Increasing MTF of any factor in the system will improve total MTF.

Dendy, P. P. & Heaton, B. *Physics for Diagnostic Radiology*, 2nd edn, IOP Publishing Ltd., 1999. pp. 203–7.

24. A. False: Scatter is produced but this is not an advantage.
B. True: High kV radiography allows a wider range of tissues to be visualized.
C. True: High kV allows a reduction in mAs and the dose is often reduced.
D. False.
E. True: Increased kV allows reduced mAs and therefore the x-ray tube is used for a shorter time.

25. A. True.
B. True.
C. False: As high kV techniques allow a shorter exposure.
D. False.
E. True.

Allisy-Roberts & Williams. *Farr's Physics for Medical Imaging*, 2nd edn, Saunders Elsevier, 2008. p. 73.

26. A. True: Tube maximum is 35Kv.
B. False: Longer since kV is low mAs must increase for an adequate image.
C. False: Normal radiography uses a 1mm focal spot, mammography uses less than 0.3mm.
D. True: 65–66cm FFD.
E. False: Moving grids are used.

Allisy-Roberts & Williams. *Farr's Physics for Medical Imaging*, 2nd edn, Saunders Elsevier, 2008. pp. 74–6.

27. A. True: A molybdenum filter removes part of the continuous spectrum.
B. False: Too high.
C. False: The anode rotates.
D. False: The AEC sits in front of both the grid and the cassette.
E. True: Combinations include MoMo, TRh, MoRh.

Electronic Learning Database, E-Learning for Healthcare, Radiology—Integrated Training Initiative (R-ITI) – www.e-lfh.org.uk
Module: 8a_072: Mammography X-ray Equipment.

28. A. True: The tissue thickness being imaged is reduced so scatter is reduced, thus reducing dose.
B. False: This is advantageous but it is not the primary purpose of compression.
C. True: See A.
D. False: The volume of the breast cannot be changed.
E. False: Maximum mechanical compression is 200N!

Allisy-Roberts & Williams. *Farr's Physics for Medical Imaging*, 2nd edn, Saunders Elsevier, 2008. pp. 75–8.

Learning Points

High KV radiography

Maximum kV is 150kV. This technique allows a wider range of tissues to be imaged on film. Skin dose is decreased as the x-rays are more penetrative. The efficiency of x-ray production is high because heat loading is reduced and exposure time is reduced. Scatter production is high so grids are less effective, an air gap is generally used instead of a grid.

High kV = Wide latitude

Advantages

- Reduced heat loading.
- Reduced exposure time.
- Reduced skin dose.

Disadvantages

- Increased scatter.
- Reduced subject contrast.

Dendy, P. P. & Heaton, B. *Physics for Diagnostic Radiology*, 2nd edn, IOP Publishing Ltd., 1999. pp. 219–21.

29. A. False: Lower keV is used with maximum tube voltage of about 30keV.
B. True.
C. False: The filter is used to attenuate most of the continuous spectrum and leaves the characteristic radiation. The filter is relatively transparent to its own characteristic radiation.
D. False: Focal spot is <0.3mm and for magnification 0.1mm.
E. True.

Sherer, Visconti, and Ritenour. *Radiation Protection in Medical Radiography*, 4th edn, Mosby, 2002. pp. 190–3.

30. A. False: Film is not used.
B. True.
C. False: Dry processing used.
D. False: Higher dose and no longer favoured for this reason.
E. True: Its use is to delineate edges of structures.

Learning Points

Mammography

Table 5.4 Mammography summary

Target	Normally molybdenum
Filter	Normally molybdenum Mo filter is used to remove most of the continuous spectrum – *not to remove the characteristic radiation*
Focal spot	<0.3mm 0.1mm for magnification
Grids	Moving
Air gap	Used
Fixed focus–film distance	65–66cm
Tube voltage	25–35kV
Screen	Single rear screen
Mo characteristic energies	17.5, 19.6kV
Rhodium characteristic energies	20.2, 22.7kV
X-ray tube	Angled for anode heel effect Beryllium window
Resolution	5 lp/mm
Dose	0.5–1mSv
Radiation risk	1/1,000,000 women screened
Main source of contrast	Photoelectric effect
For large dense breasts, breast implants, post radiotherapy	Use Tungsten target with Rhodium filter

Electronic Learning Database, E-Learning for Healthcare, Radiology—Integrated Training Initiative (R-ITI) – www.e-lfh.org.uk
Module: 8a_072 Mammography X-ray Equipment.

Learning Points *(continued)*

Anode heel effect

Mammography uses the anode heel effect by putting the thickest part of the breast (nearer the chest wall) at the cathode end where the beam is more intense.

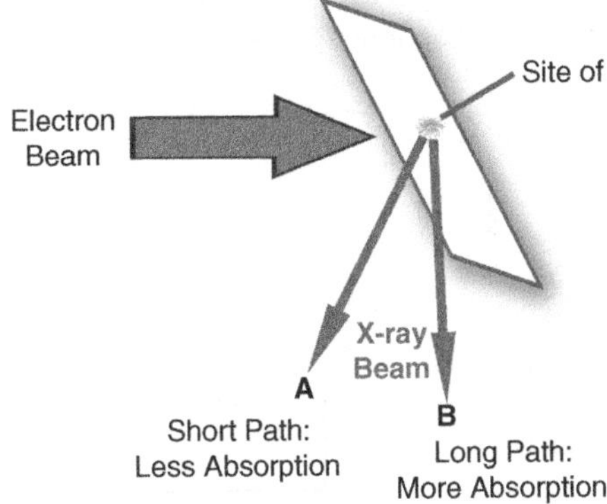
Site of Interaction
Electron Beam
X-ray Beam
A
Short Path: Less Absorption
B
Long Path: More Absorption
It is seen that x-ray beam travelling on the anode side (B) traverses more target material and therefore is more attenuated than those travelling on the cathode side (A)

Figure 5.6 Anode heel effect.

Electronic Learning Database, E-Learning for Healthcare, Radiology—Integrated Training Initiative (R-ITI) – www.e-lfh.org.uk
Module: 8a_071 Principles of Soft Tissue Imaging and Factors Affecting Dose and Image Quality.

Learning Points

Xeroradiography

This old technique doesn't use film and screen. A rigid aluminium sheet is used with a thin layer of selenium sprayed with a uniform positive charge. When exposed to x-rays, electrons are liberated in the material, which progressively discharges the positive charge. The charge remaining is relative to the amount of exposure to x-rays. Toner piles up along one side of the boundary and is depleted on the other side.

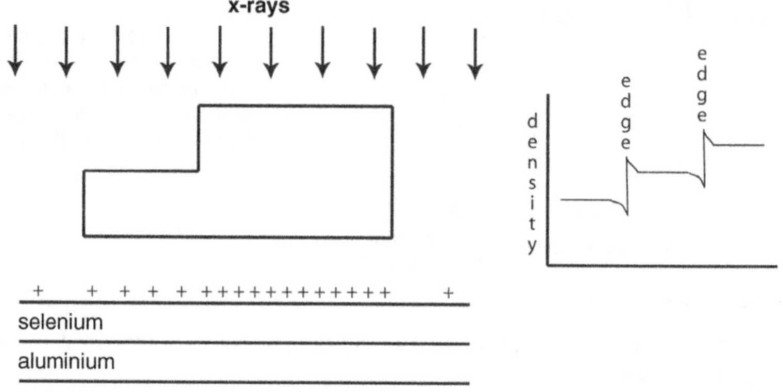

Figure 5.7 Xeroradiography

The plate is developed rapidly and dry and in the dark. The final image is transferred to paper and the plate is reusable.

Advantages

- Edge enhancement – good for looking at small structures and was often used in mammography.

Disadvantages

- Low contrast image.
- Higher dose than for film radiography, therefore no longer favoured.
- Prone to artefacts.
- Requires careful handling.

Dendy, P. P. & Heaton, B. *Physics for Diagnostic Radiology*, 2nd edn, IOP Publishing Ltd., 1999. pp. 238–41.

chapter

6

DIGITAL RADIOGRAPHY

QUESTIONS

1. The intrinsic resolution in computed radiography (CR) is limited by:

A. Pixel size.
B. Scattering of laser light in the phosphor layer.
C. Thickness of the phosphor layer.
D. Diameter of the scanning laser beam.
E. Orientation of the x-ray beam.

2. The following statements are true regarding computed radiography (CR):

A. Compared to standard image plates (IPs), high resolution image plates (HRIPs) require a lower x-ray dose to produce an image.
B. A photostimulable phosphor plate is used as the image plate (IP).
C. Absorption of an energetic x-ray photon gives electrons sufficient energy to jump from a conduction band into a valence band.
D. Electrons can decay into traps after promotion.
E. High resolution image plates have high fractional x-ray absorption efficiency compared to standard IPs.

3. In computed radiography (CR):

A. Laser light can give trapped electrons enough energy to leave energy traps.
B. The stimulated emission signal in CR has a very low intensity.
C. Photostimulable plates used in plain radiography are cheap and of single use.
D. The dose latitude (dynamic range) of CR systems is in the order of 100:1.
E. Using CR system results in a lower rate of repeat exposures.

4. The following statements are true regarding photostimulable phosphor plates (PSPs):

A. The commonly used storage phosphor comprises barium fluorohalide crystals activated with divalent europium ions.
B. A laser beam is passed across an exposed plate to read the image.
C. The image is read by continuous sampling.
D. Plate reading can take place a long while after the image is taken.
E. The density of the image depends on the exposure factors used.

5. Regarding photostimulable phosphor plates (PSPs):

A. A CR IP deteriorates over time due to laser desensitization.
B. The trapped electrons returning to their valence band release light photons of the same wavelength.
C. The modulation transfer function (MTF) is measured in line pairs per millimeter.
D. The x-ray absorption efficiency of PSP is much higher compared to that of film screen systems.
E. PSPs rarely produce image artefacts.

6. Regarding image production from a PSP:

A. The latent image stored on a plate can decay if not read promptly.
B. The speed at which the plate is read depends on developer concentration.
C. Resolution is affected by the thickness of the photostimulable phosphor layer.
D. The relative exposure versus output signal plot is a straight line.
E. Calcium tungstate is regularly used as storage phosphor in the PSP plates used in digital radiography.

7. Regarding spatial resolution of CR systems:

A. Spatial resolution of a standard CR system is significantly higher than that of competing film screen combination.
B. It depends on the diameter of the scanning laser beam.
C. It depends on the mean size of phosphor crystals.
D. It depends on the sampling interval (pixel spacing).
E. It depends on the spread of light as the laser beam penetrates the IP during readout.

8. Regarding quantum mottle in computed radiography:

A. It is directly proportional to the square of photon fluence incident upon the image plate (N).
B. It is directly proportional to the square of the fractional x-ray absorption efficiency (η).
C. It is inversely proportional to the square root of photon fluence incident upon the image plate (N).
D. It is inversely proportional to the square root of the fractional x-ray absorption efficiency (η).
E. It refers to the noise that arises from the random fluctuation in the count of x-ray quanta absorbed in the image plate to form the primary image.

9. Regarding digital radiography:

A. The charge coupled device converts photons into an electronic signal.
B. The input phosphor is coupled to the charge coupled device by fibre optics.
C. Both flat panel array detectors and charge coupled devices have dead areas.
D. Resolution on a flat panel array is limited to the width of the detector elements.
E. Image windowing can be altered after the image has been taken.

10. The following are true of analogue images:

A. The image is made up of numerous screen pixels.
B. Can easily be stored directly on a computer.
C. Can be recorded onto a magnetic tape.
D. It is used in CT.
E. Analogue images can be displayed on monitors.

11. The following are true of digital images:

A. The digital image is made up of pixels.
B. Each pixel is given a number which gives its greyscale level.
C. Each pixel is given a number which gives its point on the screen.
D. The digital image can be directly displayed on a monitor.
E. Conventionally in image display, pixels with lower values are displayed darker than ones with higher values.

12. Regarding post processing of digital images:

A. Histogram analysis of the image involves plotting the frequency of pixels against pixel values.
B. Histogram equalization is done to adjust for contrast differences in the image.
C. Vignetting is done to improve diagnostic accuracy.
D. Smoothing or blurring of features in the processed image is done by high pass filtering.
E. Low pass filtering causes enhancement of edges in the image.

13. Digital image acquisition and processing can be used by the following modalities:

A. Single photon emission computed tomography.
B. Magnetic resonance imaging.
C. Computed tomography.
D. Mammography.
E. Positron emission tomography.

14. In digital subtraction angiography (DSA):

A. Enhanced vascular structures are seen together with bony and soft tissue structures.
B. The subtraction is done using a mask image.
C. DSA does not require IV contrast administration.
D. The mA used for the DSA is the same as that used for normal screening.
E. The main advantage of frame integration is the shorter exposure time.

15. The following statements are true:

A. Images can be transmitted from plate to screen without processing.
B. Digital tomosynthesis is used to obtain images at varying depths.
C. Quantum mottle is produced by high mAs.
D. Heat blur is caused by the receptor being exposed to intense heat.
E. Histogram error artefact is caused by the use of incorrect post-processing histogram.

16. Regarding artefacts in digital subtraction angiography:

A. Misregistration occurs due to structures in the mask image and contrast image not being in the same place.
B. Misregistration can be caused by peristalsis.
C. Misregistration can be resolved by moving the mask image.
D. Misregistration can be caused by the patient's breathing.
E. Misregistration can be caused by cardiac motion.

17. Regarding monitors used for image display in radiology:

A. Thin film transistor (TFT) display screens are not suitable for use in diagnostic radiology.
B. TFT monitors are a subtype of cathode ray tubes (CRT).
C. TFT screens use less power compared to most CRTs.
D. TFTs have a smaller footprint.
E. TFT screens fare much worse compared to CRTs in detecting low contrast details.

18. Regarding solid state digital radiography (DR) detectors, the following statements are true:

A. Each pixel area contains readout microcircuitry to make it possible to directly read the image out of the detector in electronic form.
B. Fill factor (FF) of the detector is the sensitive area of the pixel / occluded area of the pixel.
C. The efficiency of signal recording is increased with increasing fill factor.
D. In general, the fill factor falls as the pixel sampling interval is increased.
E. The readout microcircuitry records light or electrical charge carriers and produces an analogue signal output.

19. Regarding greyscale resolution:

A. The greyscale resolution of a digital image is defined by the number of bits of information per pixel.
B. The term 8 bits corresponds to a choice of 8 greyscale values.
C. The term 8 bits corresponds to a choice of 64 greyscale values.
D. The term 8 bits corresponds to a choice of 256 greyscale values.
E. The term 8 bits corresponds to a choice of 10^8 greyscale values.

20. Regarding DR detectors:

A. The active matrix array (readout electronics) is manufactured from an amorphous form of silicon doped with hydrogen (a-Si:H).
B. Amorphous silicon doped with hydrogen (a-Si:H) is more sensitive to radiation damage than crystalline Si.
C. Most indirect conversion detectors use CsI:Tl (Caesium iodide:Thallium) as the scintillating layer.
D. The typical thickness of the scintillating layer is about 10 mm.
E. In the read out process, the stimulating light and the output light need to be of the same wavelength.

21. Regarding DR detectors:

A. In indirect conversion detectors, the latent image is read out one line at a time.
B. In direct conversion (DR) detectors, HgI2 is used as the x-ray scintillator.
C. The most common photoconductor used in direct conversion detectors is amorphous Selenium (a-Se).
D. In direct conversion DR detectors, a metal electrode is coated on the external surface of the amorphous selenium.
E. The metal electrode is attached to a positive bias potential of 220V.

22. The following statements are true regarding DR detectors:

A. The fractional x-ray absorption of direct conversion detectors is better than that of indirect conversion detectors.
B. Indirect conversion DR detectors offer lower patient dose for the same image quality compared to direct conversion detectors.
C. Indirect conversion detectors have higher image noise for the same patient dose compared to direct conversion detectors.
D. The modulation transfer function (MTF) of indirect conversion detectors is better than that of direct conversion detectors
E. The spatial resolution of direct conversion detectors is better than that of indirect conversion detectors.

23. Regarding DR detector artefacts:

A. Non-uniform variations in sensitivity of the x-ray absorption layer causes irregular shading across the image field.
B. Defective pixels in the active matrix array cause bright or dark spots in the image.
C. Irregular shading can be corrected by pixel correction.
D. Defects in the pixel array can be corrected by gain correction.
E. Artefacts are removed at the time of image acquisition.

24. Modification of the image greyscale using a look-up-table (LUT) might be done for the following reasons:

A. To vary the mean brightness of an image.
B. To compensate for the different intensity responses of display devices.
C. To increase the spatial resolution of small isolated structures.
D. To improve the sharpness of edges.
E. To improve the presentation of fine texture patterns.

25. Spatial feature enhancement of images using an unsharp mask algorithm might be done for the following reasons:

A. To increase the visibility of small isolated structures.
B. To improve the sharpness of edges.
C. To improve presentation of fine texture patterns.
D. To increase image contrast to improve the visibility of a subtle lesion.
E. To improve the presentation of the overall greyscale range.

26. Regarding image display:

A. In AMFP (active matrix flat panel) displays, the image is generated by scanning the phosphor screen with a focused beam of electrons.
B. A CRT display uses two sheets of polarizing material.
C. CRT monitor images are susceptible to a degradation in quality due to geometrical distortion.
D. AMFP monitor images are susceptible to contrast loss.
E. The polarizing properties of liquid crystal can be rotated in response to the magnitude of an applied electrical voltage.

27. Regarding patient dose in DR:

A. It is easy to asses whether the patient has been over- or underexposed by just looking at the display.
B. Detector dose indicators (DDIs) are special electronic devices incorporated into the detectors to measure patient dose.
C. DDIs are analogous to the optical density of films.
D. High DDI values always indicate overexposure.
E. High DDI values always indicate underexposure.

28. Regarding DICOM definitions, the following statements are true:

A. Modality worklist permits the retrieval of scheduling information for that modality and patient demographics from the radiology information system.
B. Modality push allows the modality to query PACS and to find out about previous images for the patient.
C. Modality pull allows the system to store images to PACS.
D. Print service allows the modality to print to a network printer.
E. The modality performed procedure step provides information on whether the examination in the worklist is in progress or completed.

29. The following statements regarding imaging terminology are true:

A. The modulation transfer function is the ratio of input modulation to output modulation.
B. The Nyquist criterion states that the sampling frequency must be at least twice the highest frequency present in the signal.
C. Nyquist frequency is equal to two times the sampling frequency.
D. Nyquist frequency is the maximum signal frequency that can be accurately sampled.
E. Aliasing will occur if the signal frequency is less than the Nyquist frequency.

30. In digital subtraction angiography:

A. To achieve high resolution, large focal spot sizes are necessary.
B. In modern DSA systems, it is not necessary to use the same frame as mask for each subtraction.
C. X-ray tubes with lower rating can be used in DSA.
D. Subtracted images have very high signal to noise ratio compared to non-subtracted images.
E. The image is not affected by patient movement.

31. The following are true of digital mammography systems:

A. A Digital mammography system offers a wider dynamic range compared to a film screen system.

B. The spatial resolution with direct capture method is limited by the pixel size and not to the thickness of the photo-conductor.

C. Digital mammography offers better spatial resolution than conventional film screen mammography.

D. The breast dose using a digital mammography system is higher than for the film screen mammography system.

E. Digital mammography is better than film mammography in screening women who are under the age 50.

chapter 6

DIGITAL RADIOGRAPHY

ANSWERS

1. A. True.
B. True.
C. True.
D. True.
E. True.

Allisy-Roberts & Williams. *Farr's Physics for Medical Imaging*, 2nd edn, Saunders Elsevier, 2008. p. 85.

2. A. False: A high resolution IP comprises a thinner layer of finer phosphor crystals and usually does not include a light reflection layer. HRIPs are reserved for examinations demanding high spatial resolution. High resolution imaging plates have lower fractional x-ray absorption efficiency and therefore demand a higher x-ray dose than standard IPs.
B. True
C. False: After the absorption of x-ray photons, electrons jump from the valence band into the conduction band.
D. True.
E. False: HRIPs have lower fractional x-ray absorption efficiency compared to standard IPs.

Electronic Learning Database, E-Learning for Healthcare, Radiology—Integrated Training Initiative (R-ITI) – www.e-lfh.org.uk
Module: 8a_077 Computed radiography (slides 5–6).

3. A. True: This is how the phosphor plate is read with a laser beam scanning to and fro across the plate.
B. True: The signal photons have to be collected with a photomultiplier.
C. False: The plates are expensive and can be reused.
D. False: the dynamic range of CR systems is in the order of 10^4:1 (10,000:1).
E. True: Due to the high dynamic range of CR systems, there is more consistent acquisition of images with lower occurrence of incorrectly (over or under) exposed images.

Electronic Learning Database, E-Learning for Healthcare, Radiology—Integrated Training Initiative (R-ITI) – www.e-lfh.org.uk
Module: 8a_077 Computed radiography (slides 7–8).

Learning Points

The physical mechanism that describes the conversion of x-ray energy into light in a phosphor screen is known as x-ray luminescence.

X-ray luminescence comprises two component mechanisms, which both contribute to the energy conversion and are both present (to some degree) when a phosphor screen is irradiated. These are X-ray fluorescence and X-ray phosphorescence.

- Fluorescence is used in film screen radiography.
- Phosphorescence is used in computed radiography.

4. A. True: The commonly used storage phosphor is $BaFX:Eu2+$. X stands for a specific mix of halogen atoms selected from bromine, iodine, and possibly chlorine atoms.
B. True.
C. False: The image from an IP is read by discrete sampling.
D. False: Electrons will relax to their ground states from their metastable states as soon as a relaxation mechanism presents itself. If the IP is not read in good time, the image quality will degrade.
E. False: The image density is independent of the exposure factors used.

5. A. False: The degradation of the IP is due to desensitization of the phosphor screen.
B. True.
C. False: MTF is measured in line pairs cm^{-1}.
D. False: The x-ray absorption efficiency of PSP is usually lower than film screen systems.
E. False: PSPs become worn or scratched with use and have to be replaced.

6. A. True.
B. False: Developers are not used for image production in computed or digital radiography.
C. True: A thicker phosphor layer causes more scatter, therefore reducing resolution.
D. True: Image parameters such as windowing can be altered during post processing.
E. False: Calcium tungstate was used in film screen radiography in the past.

Learning Points

Spatial resolution depends on

- IP scanning parameters:
  - Diameter of the laser beam (e.g. 100µm versus 50µm),
  - IP size and the sampling interval (pixel spacing);
- Physical construction of the IP:
  - Mean size of the phosphor crystals,
  - Thickness of the phosphor layer,
  - Presence of a light reflection or absorption backing layer;
- Other factors:
  - Scatter and re-absorption of x-ray photons,
  - Spread of light as the laser beam penetrates the IP during readout—this is known to be the dominant source of blur or unsharpness in CR imaging,
  - Digital image enhancement also affects perceived sharpness of CR images.

Allisy-Roberts & Williams. *Farr's Physics for Medical Imaging*, 2nd edn, Saunders Elsevier, 2008. pp. 83–5.

7. A. False: Significantly lower.
B. True.
C. True.
D. True.
E. True.

8. A. False.
B. False.
C. True.
D. True.
E. True.

Learning Points

$\sigma_{CR} \alpha 1/(\eta.N)^{½}$

Where σ_{CR} is the standard deviation of the x-ray quantum mottle component, N is the photon fluence incident upon the CR IP, and η is the fractional x-ray absorption efficiency.

Dendy, P. P. & Heaton, B. *Physics for Diagnostic Radiology*, 2nd edn, IOP Publishing Ltd., 1999. pp. 198–200.

9. A. True.
B. True: The input phosphor is coupled to the charge coupled device (CCD) by fibre optics to increase efficiency.
C. True.
D. True.
E. True.

10. A. False.
B. False.
C. True.
D. False: Although the acquisition is analogue, the resulting image is digital.
E. True.

11. A. True.
B. True.
C. True.
D. False: It needs to be converted by a digital–analogue converter.
E. False: Conventionally, higher value pixels are displayed darker than lower value pixels.

Allisy-Roberts & Williams. *Farr's Physics for Medical Imaging*, 2nd edn, Saunders Elsevier, 2008. p. 79.

12. A. True.
B. True.
C. False: Vignetting is the phenomenon of losing light photons at the edge of an image. It is not used as a post-processing tool.
D. False: Low pass filtering leads to the smoothing or blurring of features.
E. False: High pass filtering is used for edge enhancement.

Allisy-Roberts & Williams. *Farr's Physics for Medical Imaging*, 2nd edn, Saunders Elsevier, 2008. pp. 80–1.

13. A. True.
B. True.
C. True.
D. True: This might have been *false* a few years ago as a result of low contrast resolution of the DR systems available at that time. But due to advancements in technology, more and more digital mammography units are being set up across UK.
E. True.

14. A. False: In DSA, bones and soft tissue can be digitally subtracted.
B. True.
C. False.
D. False: The mA used is higher compared to normal screening to reduce noise.
E. False: Frame integration is a technique that was used in the past to decrease signal to noise ratio. This usually led to longer exposure times.

15. A. False: Images have to be processed before display.
B. True: Digital tomosynthesis is the digital equivalent of tomography.
C. False: Quantum mottle is produced by insufficient light photons or low mAs.
D. True.
E. True.

16. A. True.
B. True.
C. True: Assuming the movement has only been lateral. It becomes trickier if rotation has occurred or if different parts of the image have moved by different amounts.
D. True: Hence breath holding, especially during renal angiography, TIPS, etc.
E. True.

17. A. False: TFT monitors are widely used.
B. False: TFT monitors are a subtype of LCD (liquid crystal display) screens.
C. True.
D. True.
E. False: In almost all studies, TFT screens were found to be as good as or better than CRT monitors.

18. A. True.
B. False: The fill factor (FF) of the detector is the sensitive area of the pixel / overall area of the pixel (where the overall area of the pixel = sensitive area + occluded area).
C. True.
D. False: FF falls as the pixel sampling interval is reduced.
E. True: The analogue signal is then digitized.

19. A. True.
B. False.
C. False.
D. True.
E. False.

Allisy-Roberts & Williams. *Farr's Physics for Medical Imaging*, 2nd edn, Saunders Elsevier, 2008. p. 80.

20. A. True.
B. False: a-Si:H is more tolerant to radiation damage unlike crystalline Si.
C. True.
D. False: About 500 micro m.
E. False: The stimulating light and output light should be of different wavelengths (the former about 10^8 times larger).

Electronic Learning Database, E-Learning for Healthcare, Radiology—Integrated Training Initiative (R-ITI) – www.e-lfh.org.uk
Module: 8a_079 Flat panel digital radiography.

21. A. True.
B. False: Direct conversion detectors do not use scintillators.
C. True.
D. True.
E. False: 5000 Volts.

22. A. False: Indirect is better than direct.
B. True.
C. False: There is lower image noise for the same patient dose with indirect conversion detectors.
D. False: MTF of direct conversion detectors is better.
E. True.

23. A. True.
B. True.
C. False: Irregular shading can be corrected by gain correction.
D. False: Defects in the pixel array can be corrected by pixel correction.
E. False: Artefacts are removed at the time of post-processing.

Electronic Learning Database, E-Learning for Healthcare, Radiology—Integrated Training Initiative (R-ITI):– www.e-lfh.org.uk
Module: 8a_080 Processing and Display of Digital Radiography Images (slide 4).

24. A. True.
B. True.
C. False.
D. False.
E. False.

25. A. True.
B. True.
C. True.
D. False: This is achieved using LUT.
E. False: This is achieved using LUT.

26. A. False: This is how the image is produced in CRT displays.
B. False: This is a feature of AMFP displays.
C. True.
D. False: CRT monitors are susceptible to contrast loss.
E. True.

Electronic Learning Database, E-Learning for Healthcare, Radiology—Integrated Training Initiative (R-ITI) –: www.e-lfh.org.uk
Module: 8a_080 (slides 8–9).

27. A. False: DR detectors have a wide latitude and post-processing ensures that the displayed image is optimized in terms of its greyscale presentation.
B. False: DDI is determined from the signal from the plate averaged over a broad region of the plate.
C. True.
D. False: The definition of DDI is manufacturer dependent.
E. False: The definition of DDI is manufacturer dependent.

Allisy-Roberts & Williams. *Farr's Physics for Medical Imaging*, 2nd edn, Saunders Elsevier, 2008. pp. 83–5.

28. A. True.
B False: Modality push allows the system to store images to PACS.
C. False: Modality pull allows the modality to query PACS to find out about previous images for the patient.
D. True.
E. True.

Allisy-Roberts & Williams. *Farr's Physics for Medical Imaging*, 2nd edn, Saunders Elsevier, 2008. p. 88: Box 5.3.

29. A. False: Modulation transfer function is the ratio of output modulation to input modulation.
B. True.
C. False: Nyquist frequency is equal to half the sampling frequency.
D. True.
E. False: Aliasing will occur if the signal frequency is more than the Nyquist frequency.

30. A. False: As in conventional radiography, to achieve high resolution small focal spot sizes are necessary.
B. True.
C. False: The x-ray tubes used will have to be of a higher rating due to the necessity to produce multiple images rapidly.
D. False: Subtracted images usually have a low signal to noise ratio compared to non-subtracted images.
E. False: Patient movement causes movement unsharpness.

31. A. True.
B. True.
C. False. The maximum resolution achievable with a digital detector is 5–9 line pairs per millimetre which is significantly lower than that of film-screen mammography.
D. False. It is lower, mainly due to the inherently higher detection efficiency of digital detectors and the use of a harder x-ray beam at each breast thickness.
E. True. This was a preliminary conclusion from the Digital Mammographic Imaging Screening Trial (DMIST).

Pisano, et al. Digital Mammographic Imaging Screening Trial (DMIST) Investigators Group. Diagnostic performance of digital versus film mammography for breast-cancer screening. *N Engl J Med*. 27 Oct 2005; 353(17): 1773–83.
Mahesh M. AAPM/RSNA physics tutorial for residents: Digital mammography: An overview. *Radiographics*. Nov–Dec 2004; 24(6): 1747–60.

chapter 7

FLUOROSCOPY

QUESTIONS

1. Concerning an image intensifier:

A. The glass envelope contains inert argon gas.
B. The metal housing is designed to prevent stray light getting into the tube and to shield from magnetic fields.
C. The main components within the tube are the input screen, focusing electrodes and output screen.
D. The focusing electrodes are designed to channel photons from the input screen directly towards the output screen.
E. The input screen is much larger than the output screen.

2. Regarding the input screen of an image intensifier:

A. It must be perfectly flat for an undistorted image.
B. The outer layer is the input phosphor and is usually caesium iodide.
C. The inner side of the screen is the photocathode, which emits electrons when the x-ray beam hits it.
D. The input phosphor is one large flat crystal.
E. The input phosphor can pick up approximately 60% of the incoming x-ray photons.

3. The output screen:

A. Is usually 25–35mm in diameter.
B. Is a pure layer of silver-activated zinc-cadmium-sulphide.
C. Converts the electron beam into light.
D. Has an anode with a positive potential of approximately 25kV.
E. Emits light bright enough to be seen with the naked eye.

4. In the image intensifier:

A. Electrons from the photocathode are accelerated towards the output screen via a series of dynodes.
B. Approximately 100 000 light photons are emitted from the output screen for every x-ray photon detected.
C. Output is usually viewed directly by a TV camera.
D. Reduced x-ray intensity at the centre of the screen causes increased brightness at the periphery of the image.
E. The conversion factor is the ratio of luminescence of the output phosphor to the input exposure rate.

5. The electron beam in an image intensifier:

A. Is accelerated from input to output screen.
B. Is focused onto the output screen by magnets.
C. Can be distorted by external electromagnetic fields.
D. Contributes to brightness gain only through minification of the image.
E. Is re-focused when a magnified field of view is selected.

6. Brightness gain in an image intensifier:

A. Is the ratio of input phosphor brightness to output phosphor brightness.
B. Is only through minification of the image.
C. Is overall approximately 50-fold.
D. Increases with increased voltage across the intensifier.
E. Increases if the output phosphor size is increased.

7. Image magnification in fluoroscopy:

A. Requires a change in the distance between input and output screens.
B. Results in better resolution of the image than with the full field of view.
C. Does not require an alteration in exposure factors to maintain similar brightness of image compared to the full field of view.
D. Results in increased patient skin dose.
E. Is usually achieved by reducing the object to intensifier distance.

8. Quantum noise in the image produced by an image intensifier:

A. Is mostly due to thickness variation of the input phosphor.
B. Is the predominant cause of overall noise in the system.
C. Can be reduced by increasing the exposure rate.
D. Is increased if the input screen is thicker.
E. Is more likely to compromise the quality of low-contrast images compared to high-contrast images.

9. In fluoroscopy, the TV camera:

A. Converts visual information from the output screen of the image intensifier into electronic form.
B. Contains an electron beam from the cathode that is focused and directed by coils so that it scans the signal plate.
C. Contains a mesh anode that overlies the graphite signal plate.
D. Produces a voltage at the signal plate that is proportional to the intensity of light being scanned.
E. Has a resolution that is better than the resolution of the image intensifier.

10. Modern image processing:

A. Uses digital processing, including noise-reduction or edge-enhancement, by a computer prior to display.
B. Uses an automatic system to drive the film cassette into place ready for spot image acquisition.
C. May utilize fibre-optic connections between the output face of the intensifier and the camera input.
D. With charge coupled device (CCD) cameras that use amorphous silicon pixels to convert the incoming light into a digital signal, has rapid read-out of approximately 30 frames per second.
E. Eliminates the distortion across the field that is present in fluoroscopy images.

11. In a fluoroscopic examination:

A. The focus to skin distance should not be less than 45cm.
B. Using the smallest field size results in improved spatial resolution.
C. The quantum sink in the formation of the image is the output phosphor.
D. The tube is operated at a much lower tube current than in conventional radiography.
E. The maximum tube current is limited by the focal spot size.

12. Automatic brightness control:

A. Allows adjustments to be made in the brightness of the image solely by adjustment of the mA.
B. Utilizes the brightness of the central portion of the image in order to optimize the image brightness.
C. Takes as an input signal a measurement of the light intensity of the image intensifier output screen.
D. May lead to poor image quality if the x-ray field extends beyond the patient.
E. May produce an image with less quantum noise if the mAs are higher.

13. Vignetting in fluoroscopy:

A. Is more marked with less curved input phosphor screens.
B. Causes the image to be brighter centrally.
C. Can be improved by strict quality control.
D. Is due to electron loss from the periphery of the electron beam.
E. Is caused by non-uniform magnification across the intensifier tube.

14. The following statements are true:

A. Fluoroscopy dose rate at the input phosphor is 1 micro Gy s^{-1}
B. Maximum entrance surface dose should not exceed 100mGy min^{-1}
C. Skin dose may be up to 10 times higher than the dose at the input phosphor.
D. A spot image taken during fluoroscopy has a dose of 10 micro Gy per frame.
E. The Health and Safety Executive must inform if the patient dose is five times the intended dose.

15. Regarding subtraction techniques in fluoroscopy:

A. There is no need to take a mask image if energy subtraction is used.
B. There can be significant movement blur in the images produced by dual energy subtraction.
C. In digital subtraction angiography very high doses of contrast medium are required for adequate visualization of vessels adjacent to bony structures.
D. Exposure factors must be kept constant for the mask and the contrast images in digital subtraction imaging.
E. Time interval differencing can be used in cardiac imaging to produce subtracted images timed to the cardiac cycle.

16. In digital subtraction angiography:

A. An image without contrast medium is electronically added to an image with contrast.
B. The mask image is taken prior to administration of contrast.
C. The signal-to-noise ratio is increased following subtraction.
D. Post-processing using pixel shift can help eliminate motion artefact.
E. Frame integration is a form of post-processing where several frames are summed to form the final image.

17. Regarding quality control in fluoroscopy:

A. Automatic brightness control is tested with the grid.
B. Limiting resolution can be measured with a line pair phantom.
C. Contrast resolution can be tested with a Leeds test object containing varying sizes and contrasts of high atomic number material.
D. A lag of 1ms is typical for modern image intensifiers.
E. Vignetting should be less than 25%.

18. Digital flat plate detectors in fluoroscopy:

A. Utilize amorphous silicon detectors with caesium iodide scintillators.
B. Have equivalent detective quantum efficiency to image intensifiers.
C. Display more limited image contrast than an image intensifier can through a TV system.
D. Display good spatial resolution of up to 20 lp mm^{-1}.
E. Provide undistorted displayed images compared to standard image intensifier images.

19. In flat plate digital fluoroscopy:

A. Dynamic range is better than with conventional image intensifiers.
B. The image produced is rectangular in shape.
C. Image noise is reduced by using a smaller field of view.
D. X-rays are directly converted to an electrical signal without the need for light production.
E. Collimation does not affect patient dose.

20. Patient doses in fluoroscopy can be reduced by:

A. Careful collimation around the region of interest.
B. Using magnified views.
C. Low pulse rate digital fluoroscopy.
D. Using an over couch x-ray tube.
E. Digital image acquisition rather than conventional film.

21. The following statements are true:

A. The radiation exposure rate is lower for fluoroscopy than for radiography.
B. The total exposure dose for a radiograph is lower than fluoroscopy.
C. Over-table tube configurations result in increased radiation exposure for the operator than under-table tube systems.
D. The biplane fluoroscopic system uses a single image intensifier to create 2 separate images.
E. Filtration is not used in fluoroscopy.

22. Regarding collimation in fluoroscopy:

A. It increases the exposed tissue volume.
B. Collimation is usually made automatically so that it is no larger than the field of view (FOV).
C. It reduces scatter production.
D. It reduces image contrast.
E. It reduces glare from unattenuated radiation near the edge of the patient's body.

23. Regarding equalization filters:

A. They are totally radio-opaque.
B. They are the same as collimators.
C. They are also known as wedge filters.
D. They reduce glare from unattenuated radiation near the edge of the patient.
E. They are made of lead-rubber or lead-acrylic sheets.

24. The following are true regarding an image intensifier:

A. An image intensifier converts incident x-rays into a minified image.
B. An image intensifier amplifies image brightness for better visibility.
C. The input layer converts electrons into a visible image.
D. Electron lenses work to accelerate electrons.
E. All components of the image intensifier are contained within a vacuum.

25. The following are methods of dose reduction techniques:

A. Intermittent fluoroscopy.
B. Removal of grid.
C. Last image hold.
D. Image magnification.
E. Dose spreading.

26. Regarding the image intensifier:

A. It intercepts the x-ray photons and converts them into visible light photons.
B. The visible light photons converted from x-ray photons are amplified.
C. It creates a large intensification in luminance at the output screen compared with that at the input screen.
D. The image intensifier is located opposite the x-ray tube.
E. The larger the image intensifier, the higher the cost.

27. The following are artefacts in fluoroscopy:

A. Lag.
B. Vignetting.
C. Veiling glare.
D. Pincushion distortion.
E. S distortion.

28. Regarding the recording of fluoroscopic images:

A. For still images, the best resolution can be achieved using a film screen combination with a spot film device.
B. Photospot cameras allow more rapid multiple-exposure sequences at a lower radiation dose than spot film.
C. A photospot camera obtains a smaller image size than a spot film device.
D. For recording motion, cine fluorography gives the highest resolution images.
E. For recording motion, cine fluorography gives the highest dose rates.

29. Regarding digital subtraction angiography:

A. The subtraction process reduces image noise.
B. With proper calibration, quantitative data can be measured.
C. A road map cannot be used in conjunction with live fluoroscopic images.
D. To image the entire peripheral vasculature using the *stepping table technique*, the imaging gantry is fixed while the patient table moves the area of interest into the field of view.
E. To image the entire peripheral vasculature using the *stepping gantry technique*, the patient table is fixed while the imaging gantry moves the field of view over the area of interest.

30. Regarding digital subtraction angiography:

A. Between the acquisition of pre-contrast and post-contrast images, the patient is allowed to move.
B. Mask pixel shift is a technique used to re-register pre- and post-contrast images.
C. Image summation is useful when the frame rates are too slow during contrast injection.
D. Temporal frame averaging is used to decreased displayed image noise.
E. Adjustment of window widths and levels is not possible.

31. Regarding fluoroscopy:

A. Pulsed mode fluoroscopy offers much better spatio-temporal resolution than continuous mode fluoroscopy.
B. In the UK, the maximum entrance skin dose rate limit for a standard patient is 100mGy per minute.
C. Automatic Brightness Control (ABC) is the same as Automatic Exposure Control (AEC).
D. The purpose of ABC is to maintain stable viewing conditions independent of patient size, body sections, and projection angle.
E. The operator should not manually adjust collimation as this is done automatically.

32. Regarding dose to staff in the fluoroscopy suite:

A. Leakage from x-rays from tube housing is typically 5 μGy/hr at 1m distance.
B. X-rays scatter from the patient accounts for most of stray radiation.
C. Secondary scatter from structures in the room accounts for most of stray radiation.
D. X-ray scatter intensity is greater on the beam exit side of the patient.
E. At 1m from the patient, the scatter is typically about 1% of the patient entrance dose rate.

33. Regarding dose in fluoroscopy:

A. Automatic Brightness Control (ABC) keeps the image intensifier entrance dose rate the same for patients of different sizes.
B. ABC keeps the brightness of the output display constant independent of image intensifier entrance dose rate.
C. The patient entrance dose rate is reduced by increasing the thickness of a copper beam spectral filter.
D. The patient entrance dose rate is increased by reducing the fluoroscopy pulse rate from 30 to 15 frames per second.
E. Selecting zoom view increases the patient entrance dose rate.

34. Regarding the image intensifier television (IITV) system:

A. It uses optical lenses to transfer images from II output screen to television sensor.
B. The primary lens is located adjacent to the TV camera sensor.
C. A circular iris is located between the primary lens and the TV lens.
D. A circular iris aperture of adjustable diameter is normally used to calibrate the light intensity illuminating the image recording device.
E. An electronic light sensor can be mounted between the primary lens and TV lens to measure the brightness of the II image.

35. The following are examples of TV sensors used in fluoroscopy:

A. Vidicon.
B. Plumbicon.
C. Chainicon.
D. Saticon.
E. CCD solid-state sensor.

36. Regarding CCD sensors:

A. They cannot be used for serial exposure applications.
B. They are small and inexpensive.
C. They have negligible temporal unsharpness.
D. They have poor thermal, electrical, and magnetic stability.
E. They have poorer geometrical precision when compared with traditional TV camera tubes.

37. Regarding the image intensifier:

A. The degree of II amplification of an x-ray image is known as the brightness gain.
B. Brightness gain is the ratio of the brightness of the output screen compared to that of the input screen.
C. Brightness gain is the product of minification gain and flux gain.
D. Minification gain is the increase in brightness due to geometrical magnification.
E. Minification gain depends on the diameter of the input and output phosphors.

38. Regarding image intensifier (II):

A. The conversion factor (Gx) is used as a measure of x-ray II tube sensitivity.
B. The conversion factor (Gx) is inversely proportional to the luminance of output phosphor (L).
C. The conversion factor (Gx) is inversely proportional to the II entrance dose rate (X').
D. The conversion factor (Gx) can be measured using a calibrated dose rate meter and a luminance meter.
E. The conversion factor (Gx) of a modern x-ray II tube typically lies in the range of 100–300 Cds $\mu Gy^{-1} m^{-2}$.

chapter 7

FLUOROSCOPY

ANSWERS

1. A. False: It contains a vacuum.
B. True.
C. True.
D. False: They focus the electron beam from the input screen onto the output screen.
E. True.

Allisy-Roberts & Williams. *Farr's Physics for Medical Imaging*, 2nd edn, Saunders Elsevier, 2008. pp. 91–4.

2. A. False: It is curved.
B. True.
C. False: The photocathode emits electrons when light from the input phosphor hits it.
D. False: It is a 0.1–0.4mm thick layer of needle-like CsI crystals arranged perpendicular to the screen to allow for internal light reflection.
E. True.

Allisy-Roberts & Williams. *Farr's Physics for Medical Imaging*, 2nd edn, Saunders Elsevier, 2008. pp. 91–4.

3. A. True.
B. False: To stop backscatter of light and act as the anode, a very thin layer of aluminium covers the screen.
C. True: Green light is produced.
D. True.
E. True.

Allisy-Roberts & Williams. *Farr's Physics for Medical Imaging*, 2nd edn, Saunders Elsevier, 2008. pp. 91–4.

4. A. False: Dynodes are used in photomultiplier tubes. In the image intensifier focusing electrodes ensure the spatial image is preserved from input to output screen.
B. True.
C. True: A TV system results in minimal loss of information and the signal can be recorded to keep a record of the procedure.
D. False: X-ray intensity is reduced at the periphery of the curved screen, so the periphery of the image is less bright (vignetting).
E. True.

Electronic Learning Database, E-Learning for Healthcare, Radiology—Integrated Training Initiative (R-ITI) – www.e-lfh.org.uk
Module: 8a_082: X-Ray Image Intensifier.

5. A. True.
B. False: It is focused by focusing electrodes that are slightly less negatively charged than the photocathode.
C. True.
D. False: It contributes through minification gain and also amplification (flux) gain (through the increase in energy due to acceleration).
E. True.

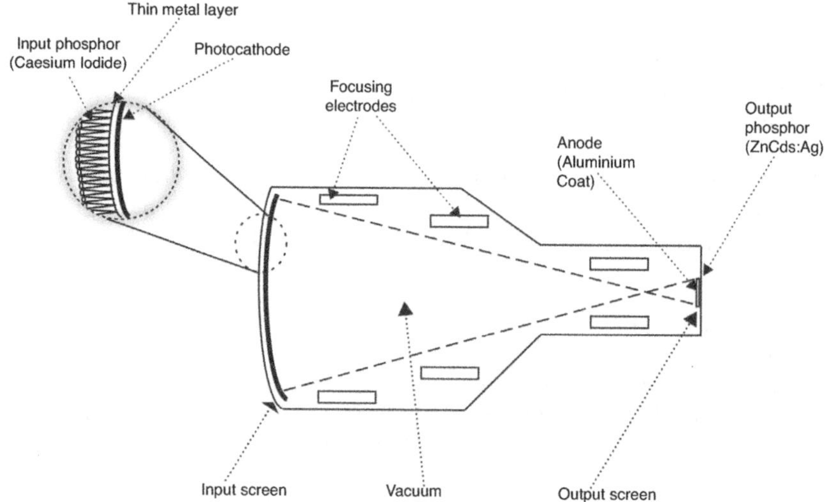

Figure 7.1 Image intensifier

6. A. False: Ratio of output phosphor brightness to input phosphor brightness.
B. False: It is through electron acceleration (flux gain) and minification gain.
C. False: It is more like 5000 (product of flux gain and minification gain).
D. True: This increases electron acceleration, therefore increases flux gain and increases overall brightness gain.
E. False: Increasing the output phosphor size reduces the minification gain and therefore reduces overall brightness gain.

Allisy-Roberts & Williams. *Farr's Physics for Medical Imaging*, 2nd edn, Saunders Elsevier, 2008. p. 93.

7. A. False: This distance is fixed. The voltage of the focusing electrodes is changed to move the electron beam crossover point nearer to the input screen, so the central part of the input image fills the whole of the output phosphor.
B. True: The TV system is one of the limits to spatial resolution, therefore the magnified image will display better resolution than the full field of view.
C. False: The magnified view has reduced minification gain, therefore reduced brightness. To restore the brightness, exposure factors must be increased.
D. True: Dose increases in order to maintain image brightness.
E. False: Although this will produce magnification, it is the re-focusing of the electron beam that produces the magnified image.

Allisy-Roberts & Williams. *Farr's Physics for Medical Imaging*, 2nd edn, Saunders Elsevier, 2008. pp. 93–4.

8. A. False: This causes screen structure noise.
B. True.
C. True: Increased dose to the input phosphor means that the signal-to-noise ratio is increased.
D. True: At any given point more photons are detected, therefore the signal-to-noise ratio is increased.
E. True.

Sherer, Visconti, and Ritenour. *Radiation Protection in Medical Radiography*, 4th edn, Mosby, 2002. pp. 177–81.

Table 7.1 Quantum noise

Increased by	Decreased by
Decreasing no of photons	**Increasing no of photons**
Increasing sensitivity of receptor (Less no of photons used to form image)	Increasing exposure rate
Increasing speed of intensifying screen (Less number of photons forming the initial image)	Increasing thickness of input phosphor (Increases no of photons absorbed – also increases blur)
Enlargement or magnification of radiograph	

9. A. True.
B. True.
C. True. Contains a mesh anode that overlies the graphite signal plate, which in turn overlies the insulated layer containing small globules of photoconductive material.
D. True.
E. False: The image intensifier can resolve 4–5 lp mm^{-1} but the TV camera has a fixed number of scan lines and will never have better resolution than the intensifier. On the TV screen the resolution may be as low as 1.2 lp mm^{-1}.

Sherer, Visconti, and Ritenour. *Radiation Protection in Medical Radiography*, 4th edn, Mosby, 2002. pp. 177–81.

10. A. True.
B. False: That was the case for older analogue image intensifiers—modern ones take digital spot images at higher mA than for fluoroscopy, but using the same camera equipment.
C. True: Traditional lens systems are now being replaced by fibre-optics for improved light collection and improved geometrical integrity.
D. True: It is more efficient converting the light directly into a digital signal.
E. False: A test object will appear curved at the edges of the image. The curvature of the input screen attempts to minimize this. However it cannot completely be eliminated even with modern image processing.

Sherer, Visconti, and Ritenour. *Radiation Protection in Medical Radiography*, 4th edn, Mosby, 2002. p. 182.

Electronic Learning Database, E-Learning for Healthcare, Radiology—Integrated Training Initiative (R-ITI) – www.e-lfh.org.uk

Module: 8a_086: Digital Fluroscopy and Flurography.

Allisy-Roberts & Williams. *Farr's Physics for Medical Imaging*, 2nd edn, Saunders Elsevier, 2008. p. 97.

11. A. True: For non-mobile equipment it should not be less than 30cm and ideally greater than 45cm.
B. True: The smaller field size is a magnified view and so has better resolution.
C. False: Overall image quality is determined at the point in the image formation process where the number of photons that contribute to the image is least. This is the quantum sink and it is the input phosphor for an image intensifier.
D. True: 25kV as opposed to around 80kV.
E. False: It is limited by patient dose restrictions.

Sherer, Visconti, and Ritenour. *Radiation Protection in Medical Radiography*, 4th edn, Mosby, 2002. pp. 177–81.

12. A. False: mA and/or kV may be adjusted to optimize image brightness.
B. True: In general the user will have centred the region of interest in the centre of the screen.
C. True.
D. True: The unattenuated part of the beam will result in a very bright portion of the image, which may lead to a much darker image when the brightness is automatically adjusted.
E. True: Although the dose will be higher to the patient.

Allisy-Roberts & Williams. *Farr's Physics for Medical Imaging*, 2nd edn, Saunders Elsevier, 2008. pp. 94–6.
Electronic Learning Database, E-Learning for Healthcare, Radiology—Integrated Training Initiative (R-ITI) – www.e-lfh.org.uk
Module: 8a_085: X-ray IITV Fluroscopy System and Automatic Brightness Control.

13. A. True: The greater curve of the input screen helps to focus the electron beam.
B. True.
C. True: Ensuring electron focusing electrodes are aligned can minimize vignetting.
D. True.
E. True: There is more magnification at the periphery of the image.

14. A. True.
B. True.
C. False: It can be 300 times higher.
D. False: 1 micro Gy per frame.
E. True: The HSE must be informed if the dose is between 3 and 20 times that intended.

15. A. True: The rapid switching between a low and high kV avoids the need for a mask image.
B. False: The high- and low-kV images are produced simultaneously.
C. False: Lower doses can be used, as there is good vessel clarity once the bones and overlying soft tissues have been digitally subtracted.
D. True.
E. True: Images are produced as the difference between images separated by a fixed interval of time, rather than all from the same mask image.

16. A. False: The image without contrast is subtracted from the image with contrast.
B. True.
C. False: Signal-to-noise ratio is reduced following subtraction.
D. True.
E. True: Retrospective summation of several frames improves the signal-to-noise ratio in the final image.

Electronic Learning Database, E-Learning for Healthcare, Radiology—Integrated Training Initiative (R-ITI) – www.e-lfh.org.uk
Module: 8a_087: Digital Subtraction Angiography.
Allisy-Roberts & Williams. *Farr's Physics for Medical Imaging*, 2nd edn, Saunders Elsevier, 2008. pp. 98–101.

17. A. False: The grid checks for image distortion. Brightness of the light output from the intensifier and TV monitor are assessed, but as deterioration in performance in the system can be masked by automatic brightness control, x-ray output must be measured directly.
B. True.
C. True.
D. True.
E. True.

Allisy-Roberts & Williams. *Farr's Physics for Medical Imaging*, 2nd edn, Saunders Elsevier, 2008. p. 99.

18. A. True.
B. True: About 65%.
C. False: Contrast resolution is limited through a TV system, but via a digital detector is much greater and makes use of the 14-bit depth that is typically available.
D. False: Resolution is better than standard image intensifiers, but with a pixel size of about 150μm, it will be about 3 lp mm^{-1}.
E. True: As the detector is flat.

Allisy-Roberts & Williams. *Farr's Physics for Medical Imaging*, 2nd edn, Saunders Elsevier, 2008. p. 101.

19. A. True.
B. True: The image displayed is the same shape as the detector.
C. False: Image noise is unaffected by a change in the field size.
D. False: Light is produced by the caesium iodide scintillator and then detected by the amorphous silicon detectors.
E. False.

20. A. True: The volume of patient irradiated is reduced and scatter is reduced.
B. False: Although the volume of patient irradiated is smaller, exposure factors are increased to compensate for the smaller minification of the magnified field of view.
C. True.
D. False.
E. True.

21. A. True: For example, fluoroscopy of a typical adult abdomen requires 45mGy/min. For an abdominal radiograph, entrance skin exposure is approximately 3mGy with an exposure time of 200ms and an exposure rate of 900mGy/min.
B. True: This is because in fluoroscopy despite having a lower exposure rate, the total exposure time is extended for the whole examination.
C. True: As the scattered radiation from the patient is more concentrated in the direction towards the x-ray tube.
D. False: Biplane systems use two separate imaging chains so that it is possible to record two projections (e.g. frontal and lateral) simultaneously.
E. False: Filtration is added to attenuate low-energy x-rays from the beam. Aluminium is most commonly used.

Schueler. The AAPM/RSNA physics tutorial for residents: General overview of fluoroscopic imaging. *Radiographics.* Jul-Aug 2000; 20(4): 1115–26.

22. A. False: It reduces the exposed tissue volume.
B. True: Although, it is often useful for the operator to further collimate the beam to the area of clinical interest.
C. True.
D. False: It improves image contrast.
E. True.

23. A. False: Equalization filters are partially radiolucent blades that are used to provide further beam shaping in addition to collimation.
B. False: They are different. See above.
C. True: They are also known as contour filters.
D. True.
E. True.

Schueler. The AAPM/RSNA physics tutorial for residents: General overview of fluoroscopic imaging. *Radiographics.* Jul-Aug 2000; 20(4): 1115–26.

24. A. True.
B. True.
C. False: That is the function of an output layer. Input layer converts x-rays into electrons.
D. False: Electron lenses are used to focus electrons.
E. True.

25. A. True.
B. True: The use of a grid increases the dose, but it is used primarily to increase contrast and image quality.
C. True: The last image is 'digitally frozen' so that the operator can look more closely at the last image without having to continually expose the patient.
D. False: This increases the patient's dose.
E. True: A reduction of the maximum skin dose can be achieved by rotating the fluoroscope but remaining centred on the area of interest and therefore the maximum dose is spread over a broader area of patient's skin.

Mahesh. Fluoroscopy: patient radiation exposure issues. *Radiographics.* Jul-Aug 2001; 21(4): 1033–45. Review.

26. A. True.
B. True: This may sound obvious but (a) and (b) are essentially two major functions of the image intensifier.
C. True.
D. True.
E. True.

Wang and Blackburn. The AAPM/RSNA physics tutorial for residents: X-ray image intensifiers for fluoroscopy. *Radiographics*. Sep-Oct 2000; 20(5): 1471–7. Review.

27. A. True: This is a persistence of luminescence after x-ray has been stopped.
B. True: This results from an unequal collection of light at the centre compared to the periphery.
C. True: This is from scattering light and a defocusing of photoelectrons.
D. True:. This is a geometric, non-linear magnification across the image that results from a magnification difference at the periphery of the image.
E. True: External electromagnetic sources affect electron paths at the periphery of the image intensifier more than at the centre and can cause the image distortion in an S-shape.

Wang and Blackburn. The AAPM/RSNA physics tutorial for residents: X-ray image intensifiers for fluoroscopy. *Radiographics*. Sep-Oct 2000; 20(5): 1471–7. Review.

28. A. True.
B. True.
C. True.
D. True.
E. True: Cine fluorography gives the highest resolution but also the highest dose rates compared with videotape recording of high-resolution TV.

Geise. Fluoroscopy: Recording of fluoroscopic images and automatic exposure control. *Radiographics*. Jan-Feb 2001; 21(1): 227-–36. Review.

29. A. False: Subtraction process increases image noise, but the perception of low-contrast vessels is increased due to the removal of distracting background tissue.
B. True: It is common practice to measure the degree of stenosis, for example.
C. False: The idea of road mapping is to provide an overlay of a static image (such as that of the vasculature) over the real-time images. In addition, 'image fade' allows the operator to manually adjust the brightness of the static vessel road map overlay.
D. True.
E. True.

Pooley, McKinney, and Miller. The AAPM/RSNA physics tutorial for residents: Digital fluoroscopy. *Radiographics*. Mar-Apr 2001; 21(2): 521–34.

30. A. False: Movement will result in a misregistration artefact.
B. True: This may help if the patient has moved between pre- and post-contrast images.
C. False: Imaging frames may occur so rapidly that only part of contrast filled vessel is captured. Summation is used so that a complete vessel segment filled with contrast is obtained within a single image.
D. True: This is done by creating an average between the current and one or more previous frames.
E. False: This can be done and is termed grey-scale processing.

Pooley, McKinney, and Miller. The AAPM/RSNA physics tutorial for residents: Digital fluoroscopy. *Radiographics*. Mar-Apr 2001; 21(2): 521–34.

31. A. True: This is particularly evident when imaging rapidly moving anatomy, such as coronary vessels in cardiac angiography or structures within the young infant.
B. True: Although in practice, a lower maximum dose rate limit of 50mGy per minute is more commonly adopted.
C. False: AEC is used in radiography.
D. True.
E. False: Manually adjusting collimation on to the clinical region of interest is good practice to reduce dose.

Electronic Learning Database, E-Learning for Healthcare, Radiology—Integrated Training Initiative (R-ITI) – www.e-lfh.org.uk
8a_085 - X-Ray IITV Fluoroscopy System and Automatic Brightness Control.

32. A. True.
B. True.
C. False: See (B).
D. False: It is much greater on the beam entrance side of the patient.
E. False: It is typically about 0.1% of patient entrance dose rate at 1m.

33. A. True.
B. True.
C. True.
D. False: Patient entrance dose rate is *reduced* by reducing the fluoroscopy pulse rate from 30 to 15 frames per second
E. True.

Electronic Learning Database, E-Learning for Healthcare, Radiology—Integrated Training Initiative (R-ITI) – www.e-lfh.org.uk
8a_085 - X-Ray IITV Fluoroscopy System and Automatic Brightness Control.

34. A. True.
B. False: The primary lens is located adjacent to the II output screen.
C. True.
D. True: The iris aperture is also used to compensate for some fall in II gain when a zoom field is selected.
E. True: This can give the real-time dose rate.

Electronic Learning Database, E-Learning for Healthcare, Radiology—Integrated Training Initiative (R-ITI) – www.e-lfh.org.uk
8a_083 - IITV Fluoroscopy Channel.

35. A. True.
B. True.
C. True.
D. True.
E. True.

All are examples of various TV sensors and differ in terms of contrast, spatial resolution, lag, and target burn resistance. Solid-state charge coupled device (CCD) sensors are superseding the traditional electronic camera tube as the preferred image recording device in modern IITV fluoroscopy systems.

Electronic Learning Database, E-Learning for Healthcare, Radiology—Integrated Training Initiative (R-ITI) – www.e-lfh.org.uk
8a_083 - IITV Fluoroscopy Channel.

36. A. False: They can be used for serial exposure applications.
B. True.
C. True.
D. False: They have excellent thermal, electrical, and magnetic stability.
E. False: They have good geometrical precision and spatial uniformity.

37. A. True.
B. True.
C. True.
D. False: It is due to geometrical *demagnification* of the image.
E. True: Minification gain = $(D_{input}/D_{output})^2$

Electronic Learning Database, E-Learning for Healthcare, Radiology—Integrated Training Initiative (R-ITI) – www.e-lfh.org.uk
8a_082 - X-Ray Image Intensifier (Peninsula).

38. A. True.
B. False: It is directly proportional to this.
C. True: Gx = L/X'
D. True.
E. False: This typically lies in the range of 10–30 $Cds\mu Gy^{-1}m^{-2}$.

Electronic Learning Database, E-Learning for Healthcare, Radiology—Integrated Training Initiative (R-ITI) – www.e-lfh.org.uk
8a_082 - X-Ray Image Intensifier (Peninsula).

16. A False: they can be used for term exposure applications.
B True.
C True.
D False. They have excellent thermal, chemical and [illegible]
E False. They have good [illegible]

17. A True.
B True.
C [illegible]
[illegible]

35. A True.
B False. [illegible]
C [illegible]
D True.
E False. [illegible]
[illegible]

chapter

8

COMPUTED TOMOGRAPHY

QUESTIONS

1. Regarding computed tomography:

A. Typical kVp value for the x-ray tube is about 80–140KV.
B. Transmitted x-ray intensity is measured by the detector.
C. It may be considered a low-dose examination in comparison to plain radiography.
D. The main interaction in CT scanning is the Compton effect.
E. The x-ray beam emerging from the tube housing in a CT scanner is significantly attenuated.

2. Regarding CT scanners:

A. Most multi-slice scanners are based on fifth generation scanner geometry.
B. An x-ray tube is mounted with its anode cathode axis perpendicular to the axis of rotation.
C. The axis of rotation is called the x-axis by convention.
D. Bow-tie filters are used to even out a beam-hardening effect.
E Fifth-generation scanners employ an electron source to produce an electron beam.

3. Regarding detectors used in CT scanners:

A. Gas detectors contain inert gases at pressures of about 1–2 atmospheres.
B. The detectors should be manufactured with identical sensitivities.
C. Pixel size is determined by the detectors.
D. The spatial resolution of the scanner is influenced by the detectors.
E. Sodium iodide crystals are the commonest detectors used in modern scanners.

4. Regarding CT scanners:

A. Third-generation scanners are more efficient in eliminating scattered radiation than first-generation scanners.
B. Tube rotation enables tube loading to be lower compared to plain radiographs.
C. The irradiated slice thickness of the patient can be regulated by detector collimators.
D. The fan beam is parallel to the anode cathode axis of the CT x-ray tube.
E. The minimum detectable contrast of CT images is <0.5%.

5. Regarding CT detectors:

A. The detectors may consist of crystals embedded in a matrix.
B. Solid state detectors are less efficient than gas filled ionization detectors.
C. Using crystals with highly efficient absorption results in a crosstalk artefact.
D. Slice thickness can be increased by coupling together the signal from adjacent detectors.
E. The detectors need to be as small as possible.

6. Regarding CT scanners:

A. Collimation of the CT scanner is fixed.
B. The most common image reconstruction technique used in modern CT scanners is filtered back projection.
C. Beam collimation happens before passing through the patient.
D. Multiple X-ray tubes are commonly used to acquire data in modern scanners.
E. Solid state detectors are more efficient than gas filled detectors.

7. Regarding CT scanners:

A. The afterglow of bismuth germinate detectors is higher compared to sodium iodide crystals.
B. The typical thickness of the copper filters used is 0.5mm.
C. The effect of scattered radiation is eliminated by using energy discriminators.
D. In fourth-generation CT design, the detectors rotate.
E. In all modern scanners, each detector has its own collimator.

8. Regarding modern CT scanners:

A. They can use thousands of detector elements.
B. Scattered radiation is controlled by detector collimation.
C. The efficiency of sodium iodide crystals is about 50%.
D. The effective dose to the patient is measured for every CT scan.
E. Ring artefacts are caused by the miscalibration of detectors in third-generation scanners.

9. Regarding image reconstruction:

A. 'Pixel' stands for 'x-ray picture'.
B. 'Voxel' stands for 'volume element'.
C. The average linear attenuation coefficient of a voxel is represented as a pixel in the image.
D. A voxel is a three-dimensional region within a scan slice matrix.
E. Star artefact can be produced by simple back projection.

10. Regarding CT number:

A. It is the same as Hounsfield units.
B. A magnification factor of 1000 or more is used in the calculation of CT number.
C. The CT number of Fat is about – 400.
D. There is no difference between the CT numbers of gray and white matter in the brain.
E. The CT number of water is – 500.

11. Regarding CT number:

A. CT number represents the linear attenuation coefficient in each pixel.
B. CT numbers of tissues vary depending on the KV and filtration of the x-ray beam.
C. It is necessary to use a CT number higher than bone to image materials that have a higher linear attenuation coefficient.
D. The CT number of air is –1000
E. The CT number of contrast is higher than that of bone.

12. Regarding CT image:

A. Image reconstruction involves a correction for the polychromatic nature of the beam.
B. A voxel is a three-dimensional region in the image display.
C. An image can only be reconstructed from data collected from a full 360° rotation of the gantry.
D. Fourier transformation can be used for image processing in CT.
E. Detector collimation controls the size of a pixel.

13. The following statements regarding CT image are true:

A. Iterative reconstruction is the most commonly used method for image reconstruction.
B. Digital subtraction is used in all CT image reconstruction.
C. The width of the x-ray beam determines the size of the voxel.
D. A voxel represents a definable region within a CT slice matrix.
E. Noise is inversely proportional to the square root of the number of photons.

14. Regarding CT image reconstruction:

A. Applying a weighting factor compensates for the difference between the size and the shape of the scanning beam and the picture matrix.
B. The weighting factor is constant throughout each complete scan.
C. The physical density of its contents is the only factor that determines the CT number of a voxel.
D. A pulse height analyser is used in CT image reconstruction.
E. A voxel is a group of four adjacent pixels.

15. Regarding helical scanners:

A. The pitch of the scanner can be defined as table-top movement per rotation multiplied by slice thickness.
B. The voxel size in the transaxial plane is determined by the matrix size and the field of view.
C. Helical scanners in general have faster acquisition times compared to single slice scanners.
D. Movement artefacts are generally lower in images obtained from helical scanners compared to single slice scanners.
E. The slice width cannot be less than the detector width.

16. Regarding image quality in CT:

A. The effect of noise is reduced by using a narrower window while displaying the images.
B. Contrast in the image is reduced by noise.
C. The effect of noise is decreased by increasing slice thickness.
D. Increasing the pixel size decreases spatial resolution.
E. Increasing the detector element size decreases the spatial resolution.

17. Regarding Image quality in CT:

A. Cupping is caused by detector malfunction.
B. The spatial resolution of CT is affected by slice width.
C. Window level determines the number of shades of grey that would be displayed.
D. Compared to film screen radiography, line pair resolution is better in CT.
E. Noise in CT makes low-contrast objects difficult to distinguish.

18. Regarding CT images:

A. Pixel size is generally about 1mm.
B. Decreasing pixel size increases the spatial resolution of CT.
C. Increasing voxel size increases spatial resolution.
D. Increasing pitch increases image unsharpness.
E. Decreasing mA decreases image noise.

19. Regarding CT scans:

A. Resolution can be improved by magnification of the subject.
B. Air is used as a negative contrast agent.
C. Iodinated contrast agents are rarely used.
D. Image quality is limited by quantum mottle.
E. Partial volume effect is reduced by using thicker slices.

20. Regarding CT artefacts:

A. Reducing beam filtration increases beam hardening artefacts.
B. Cardiac motion produces streak artefacts.
C. Geometric artefacts are caused by faulty detectors.
D. Cone beam artefact is due to beam divergence in the x-axis.
E. Ring artefacts are most commonly seen in scanners that have fixed detectors.

21. Regarding partial volume effect:

A. A thin high-contrast structure that crosses the transaxial plane at an oblique angle might disappear completely.
B. It is increased when the slices get thinner.
C. It reduces the visibility of low-contrast details.
D. A high-contrast object that is smaller than the voxel will appear larger on the image.
E. It is due to the averaging of CT numbers in each voxel.

22. Regarding CT dose index (CTDI):

A. CTDI is a measure of the radiation dose from the whole examination.
B. CTDI varies with slice width.
C. CTDI is measured in mGy cm.
D. CTDI is measured using a pencil ionization chamber.
E. CTDIvol is derived by multiplying CTDIw with pitch.

23. In helical scanning:

A. The position of the reconstructed segment can be selected retrospectively.
B. The slice width can be smaller or larger than the detector width.
C. Keeping all other parameters constant, increasing pitch reduces exposure time.
D. Keeping all other parameters constant, increasing pitch increases patient dose.
E. Keeping all other parameters constant, increasing pitch decreases resolution.

24. Spatial resolution in CT scanning is affected by:

A. Pixel size.
B. Field of view.
C. Matrix size.
D. Algorithm used.
E. Beam filtration.

25. The following statements are true regarding image noise:

A. The biggest contributor to image noise is electronic noise produced in the measuring system.
B. Quantum noise is increased by increasing the field of view (FOV).
C. Quantum noise is increased by using a larger matrix.
D. For single slice scanners, increasing the pitch increases noise.
E. For multi-slice scanners, increasing the pitch increases noise.

26. Regarding dose length product (DLP):

A. The DLP of a CT scan is calculated by multiplying weighted CTDI (CTDIw) with the total length of scan (L).
B. Conversion coefficients to derive effective dose from DLP are independent of scanner design.
C. Conversion coefficients to derive effective dose from DLP depend on body region.
D. Organs in the pelvis have a low E/DLP factor.
E. Tissues and organs in the head have a low E/DLP factor.

27. Regarding CT detectors:

A. Ionization chambers have a detection efficiency of about 40%.
B. CT detectors need to have a low dynamic range to improve resolution.
C. In modern scanners, the individual detectors need to be as big as possible to reduce scan time.
D. Bismuth germinate may be used as a scintillant in solid state detectors.
E. The overall efficiency of solid state detectors is compromised as they have to be separated to prevent light cross over.

28. The following are used for the calibration of the CT number scale of the scanner:

A. Iodine.
B. Air.
C. Water.
D. Bone.
E. Fat.

29. Regarding CT scanners:

A. Gas filled detectors are more efficient than solid state detectors.
B. The anode cathode axis of the x-ray tube is perpendicular to the fan beam.
C. The fan beam is collimated such that it is half the width of the patient.
D. The axis of rotation is called the z-axis.
E. Tube loading is much higher compared to plain x-rays.

30. Regarding CT artefacts:

A. Beam hardening is the same throughout the field of view for a given patient.
B. Tube current modulation is used to correct beam hardening artefact.
C. Compared to other metals, titanium is known to cause more artefacts.
D. Contrast agents do not produce artefacts.
E. Helical scanning is less susceptible to artefacts caused by patient motion than axial scanning.

31. The following artefacts are manifested as streaks in the image:

A. Inadequate field of view.
B. Photon starvation.
C. Motion.
D. Cone beam effects.
E. Beam hardening.

32. Regarding CT dose measurements:

A. CTDIvol is directly proportional to pitch.
B. CTDIw of the head is lower than that of the body (for the same mAs and kVp).
C. Dose length product (DLP) is inversely proportional to pitch.
D. DLP is directly proportional to the scanned length.
E. On an average, the effective dose for the head is lower than that for the body.

33. The following statements are true:

A. The effective dose is measured in mSv.
B. CTDI is measured in mGy cm^3.
C. DLP is measures in mGy cm.
D. The dose area product is measured in cGy cm^2.
E. E/DLP (DLP to effective dose conversion coefficient) is measured in mSv (mGy cm^{-1}).

34. In CT images:

A. Noise is inversely proportional to the number of photons.
B. Doubling the mA reduces the noise by a factor of 2.
C. Halving rotation time decreases noise by a factor of the square root of 2.
D. Increasing slice thickness decreases noise.
E. Pixel size is generally less than 0.5mm.

35. Regarding CT numbers:

A. CT numbers for the majority of organ soft tissues are in the range of 0–70.
B. The CT number range for lung is between –100 and –1600.
C. The CT number of blood is similar to that of soft tissue.
D. The CT number of fat is between 10 and 50.
E. The CT number of grey matter in the brain is between 35 and 45.

36. Regarding CT image:

A. The 'Filter' applied in filtered back projection is identical for all types of tissues in the same scanner.
B. In multi-slice scanning, two-point interpolation is used for image reconstruction.
C. In single slice scanning, filter interpolation is used for image reconstruction.
D. Window width represents the number of Hounsfiled Units (HU) displayed.
E. Window level represents the middle value of the number of HU displayed.

37. Regarding patient radiation dose:

A. Increasing kV always leads to an increased dose to the patient.
B. In helical scanners, reconstruction on thinner slices may increase the dose.
C. In a single slice scanner, generally the patient dose is decreased with increasing slice width.
D. mA modulation leads to a lower patient dose compared to fixed mA techniques.
E. Using a pitch of 1.5 rather than 1 leads to a dose reduction of 50%.

38. Regarding patient dose, keeping all other parameters constant:

A. Doubling mA doubles the patient dose.
B. Halving rotation time halves the dose.
C. Halving rotation time doubles the dose.
D. Doubling the pitch doubles the dose.
E. Doubling the pitch halves the dose.

39. The European guidelines on quality criteria for computed tomography (EUR 16262 EN) give:

A. A guidance on image quality and radiation dose on a generic examination by examination basis.
B. Guidance on structures that should be visible for a given type of examination.
C. A qualitative guide to the degree of clarity of structures to be expected.
D. Examples of good imaging techniques and settings.
E. Reference dose values in terms of CTDIw and DLP.

40. Regarding ECG gating in CT scanners:

A. ECG gating requires the addition of extra hardware and software to existing scanners.
B. ECG gating can only be done prospectively.
C. ECG gating always results in a lower dose to the patient compared to ungated scans.
D. ECG gating decreases image degradation due to cardiac motion.
E. In prospective gating, most of the image acquisition is done during systole.

41. Regarding cardiac CT:

A. The typical effective dose for routine cardiac CT angiography is comparable to that of abdominal-pelvic CT.
B. Dose can be decreased by increasing pitch.
C. Decreasing x-ray current during phases of the cardiac cycle is effective in reducing dose.
D. If the patient has a higher heart rate, increasing the pitch is a useful dose reduction technique.
E. Dual source CT means that one x-ray tube is used with two sets of x-ray detectors.

42. The following are effective dose reduction methods in cardiac CT:

A. Tube current modulation.
B. Reducing pitch.
C. Decreasing tube current during phases of cardiac cycle.
D. Matching the pitch to the patient's heart rate.
E. Increasing the scanning time.

43. The following statements are true of cardiac CT:

A. It requires a low temporal resolution to image the moving heart.
B. Imaging is primarily directed at acquiring images during the systolic phase.
C. Spatial resolution is not as important as temporal resolution in cardiac CT.
D. The faster the gantry rotation time, the greater the temporal resolution achieved.
E. Prospective ECG triggering acquisition reduces the radiation exposure.

44. Regarding cardiac CT:

A. In prospective ECG gating, the scanner starts at a preset point from the R–R interval.
B. The retrospective gating mode of acquisition has a higher radiation dose compared with prospective gating.
C. Multiple-segment reconstruction can result in misregistration and degrade spatial resolution.
D. Partial scan reconstruction achieves high temporal resolution.
E. Radiation dose is inversely proportional to pitch.

chapter 8

COMPUTED TOMOGRAPHY

ANSWERS

1. A. True: Typical kVp value is about 120.
   B. True.
   C. False: High dose examination. CT accounts for more than 40% of radiation from medical examinations.
   D. True.
   E. False: There is only a small loss of photon energy when the beam travels through the tube housing.

2. A. False: Most multi-slice scanners are based on third-generation scanner geometry.
   B. False: The anode cathode axis is parallel to the axis of rotation.
   C. False: The axis of rotation is called the Z-axis.
   D. True.
   E. True.

Learning Points

Table 8.1 Differences between various generation scanners

First-generation scanners	Rotate—translate
Second-generation scanners	Rotate—translate with bank of detectors
Third-generation scanners	Rotate—rotate
Fourth-generation scanners	Rotate stationary
Fifth-generation scanners	Electron beam

Allisy-Roberts & Williams. *Farr's Physics for Medical Imaging*, 2nd edn, Saunders Elsevier, 2008. p. 106.

3. A. False: The inert gases are contained at about 25atm. to increase detector efficiency.
   B. False: The detector sensitivities are calibrated during imaging.
   C. False: The computer system determines the pixel size.
   D. True: The smaller the individual detector, the higher the resolution.
   E. False.

4. A. False: Third-generation scanners produce more scatter compared to first-generation scanners.
   B. False: Tube loading is much higher compared to plain radiographs.
   C. True.
   D. False: The fan beam is perpendicular to the anode cathode axis.
   E. True.

5. A. False: CT detectors consist of single large crystals. Intensifying screens consist of crystals embedded within a matrix.
B. False: Solid state detectors have higher efficiency than gas filled ionization chambers.
C. False: Increasing the efficiency of absorption results in less crosstalk artefact.
D. True.
E. True.

6. A. False. Collimation can be changed.
B. True.
C. True.
D. False: A single x-ray tube is used. There are a few scanners that have more than one x-ray tube (currently for research only).
E. True.

7. A. False: The afterglow of bismuth germinate detectors is lower compared to sodium iodide crystals.
B. True.
C. False: Discriminating windows are used in gamma cameras.
D. False: The x-ray tube rotates and there is a ring of stationary or fixed detectors.
E. False: Only a few scanners in the market have this design feature.

8. A. True.
B. True.
C. False: The efficiency of NaI crystals approach 100%.
D. False.
E. True: Ring artefacts are caused by the miscalibration of one detector in a rotate–rotate geometry scanner. If a detector is miscalibrated, or faulty, it will record faulty information in every projection. This misinformation is reconstructed as a ring in the image with the radius of the ring determined by the position of the faulty detector within the detector array.

9. A. False: Pixel stands for 'picture element'.
B. True.
C. True: Voxel is the volume element in the scan slice matrix and pixel is its representation in the image.
D. True.
E. True.

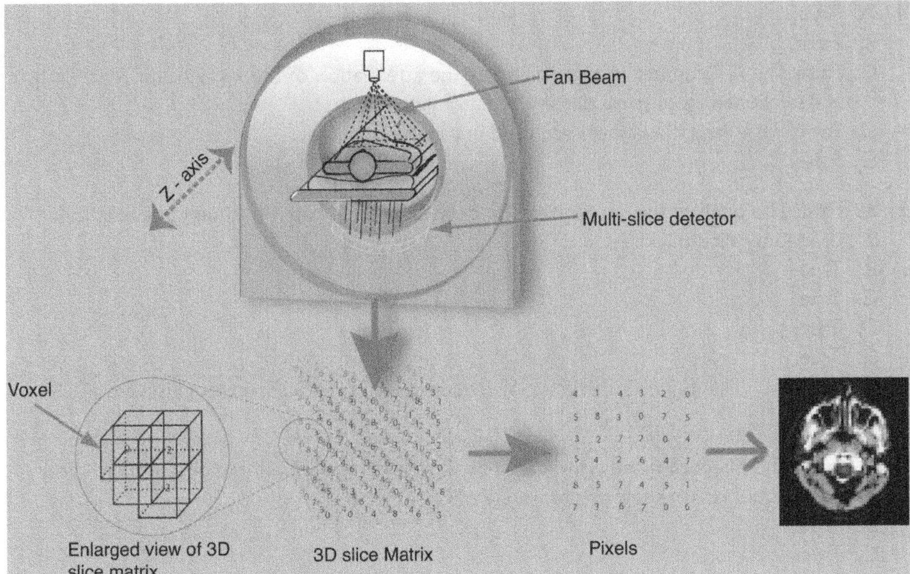

Figure 8.1 Image production in the CT scanner

10. A. True.
B. True.
C. False: The CT number of Fat is –60 to –150.
D. False: The CT number of white matter is 20–30 and that of gray matter is 35–45.
E. False: The CT number of water is 0 and that of air is –1000.

11. A. True.
B. True.
C. True.
D. True.
E. True.

12. A. True.
B. False: Voxel is a three-dimensional region in the scan slice matrix.
C. False: It is possible to reconstruct images from a reduced arc down to 180°.
D. True.
E. False: The size of an image pixel is determined by the computer program.

13. A. False: Filtered back projection is the most common method for image reconstruction.
B. False.
C. True.
D. True.
E. True.

Allisy-Roberts & Williams. *Farr's Physics for Medical Imaging*, 2nd edn, Saunders Elsevier, 2008. pp. 108–9.

14. A. True.
B. False.
C. False: The CT number is determined by the attenuation of the x-ray beam which in turn is determined by physical density and atomic number.
D. False: Pulse height analysers are used in gamma cameras.
E. False.

15. A. False: The pitch of the scanner can be defined as table-top movement per rotation divided by slice thickness.
B. True.
C. True.
D. True.
E. True.

Allisy-Roberts & Williams. *Farr's Physics for Medical Imaging*, 2nd edn, Saunders Elsevier, 2008. pp. 110–13.

16. A. False: The effect of noise is increased by using a narrower window because each grey level would represent a smaller range of CT numbers.
B. True.
C. True.
D. True.
E. True.

17. A. False: Cupping is caused by beam hardening.
B. True.
C. False: Window width determines the number of shades of grey that would be displayed.
D. False: Line pair resolution in CT is poorer than that of film screen radiography and is only about 1 lp/mm as compared to upto 15 lp/mm in film screen radiography.
E. True.

Allisy-Roberts & Williams. *Farr's Physics for Medical Imaging*, 2nd edn, Saunders Elsevier, 2008. pp. 114–15.

Learning Points

Table 8.2 CT artefacts

	Artefact	Caused by
1.	Cupping	Beam hardening
2.	Star artefact	Metal objects
3.	Ring artefact	Detector malfunction
4.	Movement artefact	Respiration, cardiac motion, patient movement

Table 8.3 Factors affecting spatial resolution

Factors increasing spatial resolution	Factors decreasing spatial resolution
Increasing sampling frequency	Increasing pitch
	Increasing pixel size
	Increasing voxel size
	Increasing detector element size

18. A. False: Pixel size is generally less than 0.5mm.
B. True: The spatial resolution of CT improves, providing all other factors like number of detectors, size of detectors, focal spot size, etc. remains unchanged.
C. False.
D. True.
E. False: Increasing mA increases the number of photons producing the image hence the image noise decreases.

19. A. True.
B. True.
C. False: Iodinated contrast agents are used regularly.
D. True.
E. False: The partial volume effect is due to averaging of the attenuation coefficient of different objects within a voxel. Using thinner slices can reduce this.

20. A. True.
B. True.
C. False: Ring artefacts are produced by faulty detectors.
D. False: The cone beam artefact is due to beam divergence in the z-axis.
E. False.

21. A. False: The thin high contrast structure that crosses the transaxial plane at an oblique angle (e.g. vessel filled with contrast) will appear larger.
B. False: The partial volume effect is reduced when the slices get thinner.
C. True.
D. True.
E. True.

Dendy & Heaton. *Physics for Diagnostic Radiology*, 2nd edn, IOP Publishing Ltd., 1999. pp. 270–1.
Allisy-Roberts & Williams. *Farr's Physics for Medical Imaging*, 2nd edn, Saunders Elsevier, 2008. pp. 115–16.
Electronic Learning Database, E-Learning for Healthcare, Radiology—Integrated Training Initiative (R-ITI) – www.e-lfh.org.uk
Module: 8a_104: Artefacts in CT Images.

22. A. False: CTDI is a measure of the dose from a single rotation of the gantry.
B. False: CTDI is constant with slice width.
C. False: CTDI is measured in mGy.
D. True.
E. False: CTDIvol is derived by dividing CTDIw by pitch.

Electronic Learning Database, E-Learning for Healthcare, Radiology—Integrated Training Initiative (R-ITI) – www.e-lfh.org.uk
Module: 8a_101: CT dose measures.

23. A. True.
B. False: The slice width cannot be less than the width of the detector.
C. True.
D. False: Increasing pitch decreases patient dose.
E. True.

24. A. True.
B. True.
C. True.
D. True.
E. False: Beam filtration does not affect spatial resolution in CT scanning.

25. A. False: Electronic noise is the least significant contributor to image noise.
B. False: Quantum noise is decreased by increasing FOV.
C. True.
D. False: Pitch does not affect noise in single slice scanners.
E. True.

26. A. False: The DLP of a CT scan is calculated by multiplying CTDIvol with the total length of scan (L).
B. False: There are differences in conversion coefficients for single and multi-slice scanners.
C. True: Conversion coefficients to derive the effective dose from DLP depend on body region and scanner design.
D. False: Organs in the pelvis have a high E/DLP factor.
E. True.

Shrimpton, Hillier, Lewis, & Dunn. *Doses from computed tomography examinations in the UK—2003 review*,(NRPB w67).

Allisy-Roberts & Williams. *Farr's Physics for Medical Imaging*, 2nd edn, Saunders Elsevier, 2008. pp. 116–17.

27. A. False: Ionization chambers had a detection efficiency of about 60%.
B. False: CT detectors need a wide dynamic range to improve resolution.
C. False: Detectors need to be as small as possible to improve resolution. Scan time is not affected by size of individual detectors.
D. True.
E. True.

Allisy-Roberts & Williams. *Farr's Physics for Medical Imaging*, 2nd edn, Saunders Elsevier, 2008. pp. 107–8.

28. A. False.
B. True.
C. True.
D. False.
E. False.

29. A. False.
B. True.
C. False: The fan beam is wider than the widest cross section of the patient.
D. True.
E. True.

30. A. False.
B. False: Tube current modulation (mA modulation) is used to correct the 'photon starvation artefact'.
C. False: Titanium causes fewer artefacts than other metals.
D. False: A high concentration of contrast agent produces streak artefacts similar to metal.
E. True.

Learning Points

CT artefacts and their causes

- Star artefacts: These are seen in the proximity of stationary high attenuating objects such as metal.
- Motion artefact: These are caused by patient movement, respiration, cardiac motion, etc. (to state the obvious!). This is due to a moving structure structure occupying different voxels during the scan.
- Partial volume effect: This is caused due to averaging of the attenuation coefficient of different objects within a voxel. Using thinner slices can reduce this.
- Ring artefacts are caused by the miscalibration of one detector in a rotate–rotate geometry scanner. If a detector is miscalibrated, or faulty, it will record faulty information in every projection. This misinformation is reconstructed as a ring in the image with the radius of the ring determined by the position of the faulty detector within the detector array.
- Beam hardening: As the x-ray beam passes through dense tissue (e.g. bone), the beam is filtered, increasing its average energy. As a result the centre of the image has lower CT numbers compared to slices without overlying dense tissue. This can be corrected using algorithms.
- Aliasing artefacts: These are caused when the sampling rate is lower than twice the Nyquist frequency. Sampling rate is limited by the hardware and tends to fall when gantry rotation speeds are increased (e.g. to reduce motion artefacts). The most common result is that sharp and high contrast structure boundaries are displayed as a lower contrast series of lines or streaks.
- Cone beam artefact: This is seen on the Z-axis in multi-slice scanners. This is caused due to an off-axis object being imaged by different detectors at different view angles.

Allisy-Roberts & Williams. *Farr's Physics for Medical Imaging*, 2nd edn, Saunders Elsevier, 2008. pp. 113 & 115.
Electronic Learning Database, E-Learning for Healthcare, Radiology—Integrated Training Initiative (R-ITI) – www.e-lfh.org.uk
Module: 8a_104: Artefacts in CT Images.

31. A. True.
B. True.
C. True.
D. True.
E. False: Beam hardening manifests as cupping artefact.

32. A. False: CTDIvol is inversely proportional to pitch.
B. False: The CTDIw of the head is generally higher than that of the body. Actual values vary according to the make and model of scanner.
C. True.
D. True: DLP = (CTDIw/pitch) × length.
E. True: The effective dose is relatively lower due to the lower radiosensitivity of the brain tissue.

www.impactscan.org/reports NRPB w67.

Learning Points

Table 8.4 CT dosimetry parameters

CTDI	Dose from a single rotation of the gantry Measured using pencil ionization chamber
$CTDI_w$	Takes into account the spatial distribution of dose within the patient in the scan plane Calculated by measuring CTDI at the centre and points around the periphery using standard head or body CT dosimetry phantoms $CTDI_w = 1/3 CTDI_{centre} + 2/3 CTDI_{average\_periphery}$
$CTDI_{vol}$	$CTDI_w$ / Pitch
DLP	$CTDI_{vol}$ × total scan length (L)
(or for single slice scanners)	$CTDI_w$ × total no of acquired slices (N) × Thickness of each slice (T)
E (Effective dose)	Derived from DLP using various published data sources or special computer programs
W_T	Tissue weighting factor

www.impactscan.org/reports NRPB w67.
Allisy-Roberts & Williams. *Farr's Physics for Medical Imaging*, 2nd edn, Saunders Elsevier, 2008. pp. 116–17.
Electronic Learning Database, E-Learning for Healthcare, Radiology—Integrated Training Initiative (R-ITI) – www.e-lfh.org.uk
Module: 8a_108: CT Image Quality and Dose: trade offs and optimisation.

33. A. True.
B. False: CTDI is measured in mGy.
C. True.
D. True.
E. True.

34. A. False: Noise is inversely proportional to the square root of the number of photons.
B. False: Doubling the mA reduces the noise by a factor of the square root of 2.
C. False: Halving rotation time increases noise by a factor of the square root of 2.
D. True.
E. True.

Allisy-Roberts & Williams. *Farr's Physics for Medical Imaging*, 2nd edn, Saunders Elsevier, 2008. pp. 114–16.

35. A. True.
B. False: It is between –100 and –900.
C. True.
D. False: It is between –60 and –150.
E. True.

Learning Points

Table 8.5 CT numbers

Soft tissue, blood	0 to 70
Lung	–100 to –900
Fat	–60 to –150
Grey matter	35 to 45
White matter	20 to 30
Bone	500 to 1500
Air	–1000

36. A. False: The filter can be changed depending on the type of tissue being scanned.
B. False: Filer interpolation is used for image reconstruction in multi-slice scanning.
C. False: Two point interpolation is used for image reconstruction in single slice scanning.
D. True.
E. True.

37. A. False: Decreasing the mA can offset the increase in dose due to the higher KV setting. In some instances, this can lead to a lower patient dose without any increase in the image noise.
B. True: Reconstruction on thinner slices increases noise and this is compensated by increasing mAs, and thus the dose may be increased.
C. False: In single slice scanners, the patient dose is generally independent of slice width.
D. True.
E. False: Using a pitch of 1.5 leads to a dose reduction of 33%.

38. A. True.
B. True.
C. False.
D. False.
E. True.

39. A. True.
B. True.
C. True.
D. True.
E. True.

Dose is directly proportional to mAs and inversely proportional to pitch.

www.drs.dk/guidelines/ct/quality/

Electronic Learning Database, E-Learning for Healthcare, Radiology—Integrated Training Initiative (R-ITI) – www.e-lfh.org.uk

Module: 8a_108: CT Image Quality and Dose: trade offs and optimisation.

40. A. True.
B. False: ECG gating can be done prospectively or retrospectively.
C. False: There is no dose reduction in retrospective gating.
D. True.
E. False: Most of the image acquisition is done during diastole.

Electronic Learning Database, E-Learning for Healthcare, Radiology—Integrated Training Initiative (R-ITI) – www.e-lfh.org.uk
Module: 1a_006: Normal Cardiac CT.

41. A. True. This is in the region of 7–13 mSv.
B. True.
C. True: Images acquired during these phases are of lower quality and therefore deemed to be of less value for interpretation.
D. True: This is a useful feature of dual-source cardiac CT where linking pitch to a patient's heart rate can effectively reduce the dose and also obviate the need for a heart rate lowering drug such as beta-blockers.
E. False: It is 2 sets of x-ray tubes and 2 sets of x-ray detectors.

Cody & Mahesh. AAPM/RSNA physics tutorial for residents: Technologic advances in multidetector CT with a focus on cardiac imaging. *Radiographics.* Nov–Dec 2007; 27(6): 1829–37. Review.

42. A. True: This involves lowering the tube current as x-rays crosses over certain areas of the body.
B. False: Increasing pitch reduces dose.
C. True: Dose reduction of up to 50% has been achieved using this.
D. True.
E. False: Scanning time is kept to a minimum to minimize dose.

Cody & Mahesh. AAPM/RSNA physics tutorial for residents: Technologic advances in multidetector CT with a focus on cardiac imaging. *Radiographics.* Nov–Dec 2007; 27(6): 1829–37. Review.

43. A. False: In fact, the primary challenge of imaging a beating heart in a system is to have a high temporal resolution.
B. False: It is the diastolic phase as this is the most quiescent part of the cardiac cycle.
C. False: It is just as important as one must be able to resolve fine structures such as the coronary artery segments.
D. True.
E. True: This is because the projection data are acquired for short periods and not throughout the heart cycle.

Mahesh & Cody. Physics of cardiac imaging with multiple-row detector CT. *Radiographics.* Sep–Oct 2007; 27(5): 1495–509. Review.

44. A. True.
B. True: This is because data are acquired continuously during the cardiac cycle and data from ECG monitoring are retrospectively used for image reconstruction.
C. True: This is one of the limitations of the multiple-segment reconstruction approach.
D. False: This is one of the major limitations of partial scan reconstruction and is due to the gantry rotation time. Higher temporal resolution is achieved with the multiple-segment reconstruction approach.
E. True.

Mahesh and Cody. Physics of cardiac imaging with multiple-row detector CT. *Radiographics.* Sep–Oct 2007; 27(5): 1495–509. Review.

chapter 9

NUCLEAR MEDICINE

QUESTIONS

1. **Concerning nuclear stability:**

   A. Stable lighter nuclei contain nearly equal numbers of protons and neutrons.
   B. Stable heavier nuclei contain greater proportion of protons than neutrons.
   C. Isotopes have the same number of protons, chemical, and metabolic properties.
   D. Isotopes have different number of neutrons, mass number, density, and physical properties.
   E. Unstable radioactive nuclei have proton or neutron excess or deficit and decay until they become stable.

2. **Concerning radionuclides:**

   A. All radionuclides used for medical imaging are produced artificially.
   B. Molybdenum-99 (^{99}Mo) is unstable as it is neutron deficient.
   C. Fluorine-18 (^{18}F) is unstable due to excess of neutron.
   D. ^{99}Mo can be extracted from the spent fuel rods of nuclear reactors.
   E. Gallium-68 (^{68}Ga) is produced from a germanium-68 (^{68}Ge) generator.

3. **The following are true of radioactive decay:**

   A. In β^- decay, the atomic number of the daughter nucleus increases by 1.
   B. In β^+ decay, the atomic mass of the daughter nucleus increases by 1.
   C. The majority of the metastable radionuclides undergo isomeric transition.
   D. In electron capture, the atomic mass decreases by 1.
   E. Radionuclides which undergo internal conversion can emit both photoelectrons and characteristic x-rays.

4. **Concerning radioactive emissions:**

   A. Gamma rays emitted for a given radionuclide have a few specific energies which are characteristic of that nuclide.
   B. Internal conversion is when emitted gamma rays do not leave the atom and are photoelectrically absorbed by the K-shell.
   C. Beta radiation emits at specific energies like gamma rays.
   D. The most energetic beta rays only have a range of a few millimetres in tissue.
   E. A positron combines with another positive electron to undergo annihilation to emit two photons of 511keV travelling in opposite directions.

5. The following are true of positron emitters:

A. They are produced in a cyclotron.
B. Upon decay they emit a positive beta particle which combines with a nearby negative electron.
C. Positron annihilation emits two gamma photons of 511keV.
D. The two photons of annihilation radiation are emitted 90 degrees to each other.
E. They may be used in positron emission tomography (PET) imaging.

6. The following are true of radioactive decay:

A. It is a deterministic process governed by the laws of chance.
B. It is possible to predict the next disintegration within a sample of unstable nuclei.
C. It is possible to predict the reduction of radioactivity in a given time interval.
D. The decay rate is measured in the SI unit of millisievert (mSv).
E. The count rate measured by a radiation detector is less than the actual radioactivity.

7. Concerning the effective half-life (t_{eff}):

A. It is dependent of the biological half-life (t_{biol}) of the radiopharmaceutical.
B. It is independent of the physical half-life (t_{phys}) of the radiopharmaceutical.
C. It is the same in everyone for a given radiopharmaceutical.
D. It is not affected by the patient's renal function.
E. The effective half-life is always less than the biological half-life or the physical half-life.

8. Ideal properties of radiopharmaceuticals:

A. A physical half-life as short as possible.
B. It localizes largely and quickly to the tissues of diagnostic interest.
C. A pure gamma emitter with energy emission greater than 300keV.
D. It is easily made and readily available at the hospital site.
E. It emits gamma radiation only.

9. Desirable properties of radioactive nuclei:

A. To decay to a stable daughter product or at least one with a very long half-life.
B. To emit gamma rays with energy greater than 300KeV.
C. Attaches easily and firmly to the pharmaceutical with no effect on its metabolism.
D. High radioactive concentration in terms of high concentration per unit volume.
E. Delayed elimination from the body with an effective half-life as long as possible.

10. The following statements are true of Technetium-99m:

A. It is produced in a generator.
B. It emits gamma rays principally of 0.140MeV.
C. It has a physical half-life of 6 days.
D. It is a daughter product of the parent radionuclide ^{131}I.
E. It is a product of electron capture decay.

11. Regarding a Technetium generator:

A. The generator is shielded with lead or depleted uranium.
B. The parent ^{131}I is absorbed within the exchange column of aluminium beads.
C. In transient equilibrium, the daughter and the parent appear to decay together with the half-life of the parent.
D. Technetium is eluted with sterile water.
E. The lead shielding and the metal container are reusable.

12. The following are true of Fluorine-18:

A. It is the most commonly used PET radionuclide.
B. It has a half-life of 6 hours.
C. It is produced in a nuclear reactor.
D. It is commonly use in oncological imaging.
E. It has a neutron deficit.

13. Half-lives of radionuclides:

A. Krypton-81m (^{81}Kr^{m}) has a half-life of 13 minutes.
B. Fluorine-18 (^{18}F) has a half-life of 110 minutes.
C. Technetium-99m (^{99}Tc^{m}) has a half-life of 6 days.
D. Molybdenum-99 (^{99}Mo) has a half-life of 67 hours.
E. Technetium-99 (^{99}Tc) has a half-life of 200 days.

14. Radionuclides and their uses:

A. Iodine-123 (^{123}I) labelled to hippuran is used for renal studies.
B. Xenon-133 (^{133}Xe) is used in lung ventilation imaging.
C. Krypton-81m (^{81}Kr^{m}) is used for pulmonary ventilation studies.
D. Gallium-68 (^{68}Ga) is used to detect tumours and abscesses.
E. Thallium-201 (^{201}Th) is used in myocardial perfusion imaging.

15. Gamma camera collimators:

A. In a parallel hole collimator, the field of view and the in-air sensitivity are the same at all distances.

B. A divergent hole collimator obtains a larger field of view and magnifies the image.
C. A convergent hole collimator minifies the image when a small field of view is acquired.
D. Both the divergent hole and convergent hole collimators suffer from geometric distortion with deterioration of spatial resolution at the edge of the field.
E. A pinhole collimator produces magnified and inverted images.

16. Regarding the gamma camera crystal:

A. The crystal is made of caesium iodide and activated with a trace of thallium.
B. It is composed of multiple small crystals.
C. It emits approximately 5000 light photons when struck by a gamma photon.
D. A flat transparent light guide can maximize transfer of light from the crystal to the photomultiplier.
E. It is robust and waterproof.

17. Concerning the gamma camera:

A. Spatial resolution improves by rejecting scattered gamma rays.
B. The typical energy window is ±10% of the photopeak.
C. Two radionuclides can be imaged simultaneously.
D. The stored digital image can be manipulated.
E. Digital cameras do not require photomultiplers.

18. In a gamma camera:

A. The purpose of the collimator is to remove scattered radiation.
B. The purpose of the pulse height analyser is to filter out scattered radiation.
C. The spatial resolution is comparable to that of a CT scanner.
D. The photomultiplier tubes amplify the signal by a series of dynodes.
E. Variation in the image of a uniform source is caused mainly by variations in the thickness of the NaI (Tl) crystal.

19. The spatial resolution of the gamma camera is affected by:

A. The thickness of the crystal.
B. The diameter of the hole of the collimator.
C. The length of the hole of the collimator.
D. The count rate.
E. The number of photomultiplier tubes.

20. Quality control for the gamma camera:

A. Spatial resolution is assessed by using a flood field phantom.
B. Uniformity of field is assessed by imaging a line source.
C. Typical system uniformity is 20%.
D. Intrinsic resolution is better than the system resolution.
E. A cracked crystal will not show as a defect.

21. In single-photon emission computed tomography (SPECT):

A. It consists of a gamma camera with a collimator rotating around a patient on a couch.
B. The camera rotates continuously to acquire images.
C. It requires fewer counts than conventional static imaging.
D. The same number of counts can be acquired in half the time by using a double headed camera.
E. Sensitivity decreases when a double- or tripled-headed camera is used.

22. Advantages of SPECT over planar imaging:

A. It has the potential to correct for attenuation.
B. There is an increase in spatial resolution.
C. There is an increase in contrast.
D. There is a decrease in noise.
E. It has fewer equipment related artefacts.

23. In SPECT:

A. Filtered back projection may be used in image formation.
B. Iterative reconstruction produces fewer artefacts and can correct attenuation more accurately than filtered back projection.
C. Superimposition of overlying structures cannot be resolved.
D. Reconstruction can be performed through any plane.
E. Planar views are reconstructed to form a 3D image.

24. SPECT image resolution can be improved by:

A. Using a 128 × 128 matrix compared to a 64 × 64 matrix.
B. Increasing the administered activity of a radiopharmaceutical.
C. Using a low resolution collimator.
D. Using a smooth reconstruction filter.
E. By not reducing noise with a mathematical filter.

25. The following are necessary to perform SPECT:

A. A triple-headed camera.
B. A camera system capable of rotating around the patient.
C. A radionuclide which emits monoenergetic gamma photon energy only.
D. A radiopharmaceutical specifically designed for use with SPECT.
E. A radiopharmaceutical whose distribution within the patient is fixed.

26. In positron emission tomography (PET):

A. PET images can give functional and physiological information.
B. PET images can be fused with CT images to allow location and visualization of such information within the patient's anatomy.
C. Positrons are coincidentally detected.
D. PET imaging is based on detecting an annihilation photon to locate the source of radioactivity within the patient.
E. Annihilation photons have energy of 0.51MeV.

27. Concerning PET:

A. Most commonly used positron emitter in PET is ^{18}F.
B. Annihilation photons are detected by a ring of detectors.
C. Scintillation detectors may be made from lutetium oxyorthosilicate.
D. ^{68}Ga and ^{82}Rb are also used in PET imaging.
E. PET imaging can be combined with MRI images to assist the location of radioactivity within the patient's body.

28. Ideal properties of PET scintillation detectors:

A. Good energy resolution.
B. High detection efficiency.
C. A very short scintillation decay time.
D. High effective atomic number and physical density.
E. High relative light output.

29. Advantages of PET over SPECT:

A. Collimators are not required for PET.
B. Spatial resolution is superior to SPECT.
C. Image noise is less than SPECT.
D. Radiation dose to patient is markedly reduced compared to SPECT.
E. ^{18}F has a shorter half-life than ^{99}Tc^{m}.

30. In radionuclide imaging the radiation dose to the patient is:

A. Independent of the emitted energy of the gamma rays.
B. Inversely proportional to the administered radioactivity.
C. Independent of the physical half-life of the radiopharmaceutical.
D. The effective dose is measured in megabecquerels.
E. Dependent on the image acquisition time and the number of acquisitions.

31. The absorbed dose increases in proportion to:

A. The activity administered to the patient.
B. The fraction taken up by the organ.
C. The effective half-life of the activity in the organ.
D. The energy of the gamma radiation emitted from decay.
E. The renal excretion rate.

32. The effective dose in nuclear medicine based on UK ARSAC DRLs:

A. Is 5mSv for a bone SPECT scan.
B. Is 50mSv for a ^{201}Th heart scan.
C. Is up to 2mSv for renal studies.
D. Is 8mSv for a brain scan.
E. Is up to 2mSv for lung scans.

33. In nuclear medicine:

A. The ideal radionuclide emits both gamma and beta radiation.
B. Lead aprons are effective and should be worn if gamma ray energies are greater than 140keV.
C. Not all radioactive waste must be disposed of by a specialist waste contractor.
D. The photoelectric effect predominates when the photon energy is above 2MeV.
E. All radioactive administrations are contraindicated in women who are breastfeeding.

34. Concerning the Medicines (Administration of Radioactive Substances) Regulations (MARS) 1978:

A. An ARSAC certificate must be obtained for all procedures which use radionuclides.
B. An ARSAC licence should be obtained by all employees working in nuclear medicine.
C. The ARSAC clinical licences are valid for 5 years.
D. The ARSAC research licences are valid for 2 years.
E. A licence covers all work involving radionuclides within the hospital.

35. Concerning the Medicines (Administration of Radioactive Substances) Regulations (MARS) 1978:

A. The application for an ARSAC licence must be signed by a Radiation Protection Advisor.
B. There must be adequate scientific support in order for an ARSAC licence to be granted to an applicant.
C. The ARSAC certificate is issued by the Department of Health.
D. It is the employer's responsibility to ensure relevant clinicians possess an ARSAC licence.
E. It is the responsibility of the ARSAC licence holder to discharge a radioactive patient with the appropriate advice and hence protect the safety of the public.

36. Regarding the Radioactive Substances Act 1993:

A. It controls the accumulation, storage, and disposal of radioactive waste.
B. It is enforced by the Environment Agency.
C. Hospitals are exempted of registration under the Radioactive Substance Act 1993 for keeping any given amount of radioactive substance.
D. Once a hospital is registered under the Radioactive Substance Act 1993, there is no stipulation or enforcement on the methods of radioactive waste disposal.
E. All hospitals using radioactive substances are subjected to strict disposal limits for radioactive substances.

37. Disposal methods of radioactive waste:

A. Gas can be disposed by venting it to the atmosphere.
B. Aqueous liquid diluted with water can be disposed into the sewers.
C. Organic liquid must be disposed to an authorized contractor.
D. Solid waste must be disposed to authorized incinerators or waste contractors.
E. Contaminated clothing and bedding is bagged and securely stored until the activity is sufficiently decayed for release to the laundry.

38. Precautions in handling radionuclides:

A. Internal radiation occurs from accidental ingestion or inhalation of radionuclide.
B. Patients containing radioactivity are not a source of external radiation.
C. Personal protection should be made by distance, shielding, and time.
D. 2.5mm lead aprons are effective in providing adequate radiation protection when manipulating radiopharmaceuticals.
E. Dose reduction is achieved by using forceps and syringe shields when handling radionuclides.

39. Precautions and safety measures in nuclear medicine:

A. Patient dose from a bone scan injection is reduced by encouraging high oral intake of water and by frequent micturation.
B. Children are given radiopharmaceuticals of higher activity than adults due to their increased metabolism in order to achieve an adequate diagnostic image.
C. Female patients should avoid conception for a given period after the administration of a radionuclide with a long half-life.
D. Examinations resulting in a foetal dose greater than 10mSv should be avoided in pregnant patients.
E. Cessation of breast feeding is not necessary when lactating mothers are given therapeutic doses of Iodine-131.

40. Concerning nuclear medicine:

A. All doses must be as low as reasonably practicable (ALARP).
B. Diagnostic reference levels are equivalent to dose limits.
C. Diagnostic reference levels may be exceeded in tall obese patients.
D. Diagnostic reference levels are produced by Ionising Radiation Regulations 1999.
E. Organ dose can be calculated by the Medical Internal Radiation Dose (MIRD) scheme.

chapter 9

NUCLEAR MEDICINE

ANSWERS

1. A. True.
B. False: Stable heavier nuclei contain greater proportion of neutrons.
C. True.
D. True.
E. True.

Allisy-Roberts & Williams. *Farr's Physics for Medical Imaging*, 2nd edn, Saunders Elsevier, 2008. pp. 121–46.

2. A. True.
B. False: ^{99}Mo is made by addition of neutron to ^{98}Mo in a nuclear reactor hence it is unstable with an excess of neutron (^{98}Mo + n $\rightarrow$ ^{99}Mo).
C. False: ^{18}F is made in a cyclotron by an additional proton being forced into the stable nucleus of ^{18}O which in return knocks out a neutron hence making the nucleus neutron deficient (^{18}O + p $\rightarrow$ ^{18}F + n).
D. True: ^{238}U $\rightarrow$ ^{99}Mo + other fission by products.
E. True: ^{68}Ga is a daughter product of ^{68}Ge.

Powsner & Powsner. *Essential Nuclear Medicine Physics*, 2nd edn, Blackwell Publishing, 2006. pp. 29–36.

3. A. True: In β^- decay, the atomic number increases by 1 and the atomic mass remains unchanged in the daughter nucleus.
B. False: In β^+ decay, the atomic number decreases by 1 and the atomic mass remains the same in the daughter nucleus.
C. True.
D. False: In electron capture, the atomic number reduces by 1 whilst the atomic mass remains unchanged in the daughter nucleus.
E. True: Examples of such radionuclides are iodine-123 and iodine-125.

Allisy-Roberts & Williams. *Farr's Physics for Medical Imaging*, 2nd edn, Saunders Elsevier, 2008. pp. 121–46.
Electronic Learning Database, E-Learning for Healthcare, Radiology—Integrated Training Initiative (R-ITI) – www.e-lfh.org.uk
Module: 8a_109: Radionuclide Imaging Overview.

4. A. True.
B. True.
C. False: Beta rays emit a continuous spectrum of energies up to its maximum energy.
D. True.
E. False: Positive beta particle combines with a negative electron to undergo annihilation.

Powsner & Powsner. *Essential Nuclear Medicine Physics*, 2nd edn, Blackwell Publishing, 2006. pp. 20–8.

5. A. True.
B. True.
C. True.
D. False: They are emitted simultaneously and in practically opposite directions to each other.
E. True.

Allisy-Roberts & Williams. *Farr's Physics for Medical Imaging*, 2nd edn, Saunders Elsevier, 2008. pp. 121–46.
Electronic Learning Database, E-Learning for Healthcare, Radiology—Integrated Training Initiative (R-ITI) – www.e-lfh.org.uk
Module: 8a_109: Radionuclide Imaging Overview.

6. A. False: It is a stochastic process governed by the laws of chance.
B. False: It is impossible to predict the next disintegration in a given sample.
C. True.
D. False: The rate of decay is measured in becquerel (Bq) where 1Bq is equivalent to 1 disintegration per second.
E. True: A sufficient proportion of the rays usually miss the detector or it may pass through undetected hence the count rate is less than the activity.

Powsner & Powsner. *Essential Nuclear Medicine Physics*, 2nd edn, Blackwell Publishing, 2006. pp. 29–36.

Learning Points

Half-life

- Physical half-life ($1/t_{phys}$) is the time taken for a radionuclide activity to decay to half its original value.
- Biological half-life ($1/t_{biol}$) is the time taken to excrete half the activity from the patient.
- Effective half-life ($1/t_{eff}$) is calculated as follows:

$$1/t_{eff} = 1/t_{phys} + 1/t_{biol}$$

The effective half-life is shorter than either the biological or the physical half-lives.

7. A. True: $1/t_{eff} = 1/t_{phys} + 1/t_{biol}$
B. False.
C. False: The metabolic process of eliminating and excreting radiopharmaceutical varies between everybody.
D. False: Renal function affects the t_{biol} hence in turn it affects the t_{eff}.
E. True.

Allisy-Roberts & Williams. *Farr's Physics for Medical Imaging*, 2nd edn, Saunders Elsevier, 2008. pp. 124–5.

8. A. False: The half-life should be suitable for the examination.
   B. True.
   C. False: It should be a pure gamma emitter but with energy emission between 50–300keV.
   D. True.
   E. True: Hence scatter can be eliminated by energy discrimination with a pulse height analyser.

Allisy-Roberts & Williams. *Farr's Physics for Medical Imaging*, 2nd edn, Saunders Elsevier, 2008. pp. 125–28.
Electronic Learning Database, E-Learning for Healthcare, Radiology—Integrated Training Initiative (R-ITI) – www.e-lfh.org.uk
Module: 8a_110: Radiopharmaceuticals.

9. A. True.
   B. False: An ideal energy emission is around 150KeV where it is high enough to exit the patient but low enough to be collimated and detected.
   C. True.
   D. True.
   E. False: An ideal radiopharmaceutical should be eliminated from the body with an effective half-life as long as the duration of the examination in order to reduce the dose to the patient.

Learning Points

Radionuclides

Table 9.1 Radionuclides

	Technetium 99m	Fluorine 18
Usage	In 90% of all radionuclide imaging	Most commonly used radionuclide in PET
Energy emission	Pure gamma rays emitter 140keV	Positions (B^+) on annihilation 2 × 511keV gamma photons
Half-life	6 hours	110 minutes
Decay production from	Molybdenum-99	Oxygen-18
Derived from	Generator	Cyclotron

10. A. True.
   B. True.
   C. False: It has a half-life of 6 hours.
   D. False: It is a daughter product of the parent radionuclide ^{99}Mo.
   E. False: ^{99}Mo undergoes beta decay to produce the daughter radionuclide of ^{99m}Tc.

Allisy-Roberts & Williams. *Farr's Physics for Medical Imaging*, 2nd edn, Saunders Elsevier, 2008. p. 126.

11. A. True.
B. False: The parent radionuclide is ^{99}Mo.
C. True.
D. False: It is eluted with sterile saline solution.
E. True.

Allisy-Roberts & Williams. *Farr's Physics for Medical Imaging*, 2nd edn, Saunders Elsevier, 2008. p. 126.

12. A. True.
B. False: It has a half-life of 110 minutes.
C. False: It is produced in a cyclotron.
D. True.
E. True.

Electronic Learning Database, E-Learning for Healthcare, Radiology—Integrated Training Initiative (R-ITI) – www.e-lfh.org.uk
Module: 8a_110: Radiopharmaceuticals.

13. A. False: $^{81}Kr^{m}$ has a half-live of 13 seconds.
B. True.
C. False: $^{99}Tc^{m}$ has a half-life of 6 hours.
D. True.
E. False: Technetium-99 (^{99}Tc) has a half-life of 200 000 years.

Electronic Learning Database, E-Learning for Healthcare, Radiology—Integrated Training Initiative (R-ITI) – www.e-lfh.org.uk
Module: 8a_110: Radiopharmaceuticals.

14. A. True.
B. True.
C. True.
D. True.
E. True.

Allisy-Roberts & Williams. *Farr's Physics for Medical Imaging*, 2nd edn, Saunders Elsevier, 2008. p. 127.

Learning Points

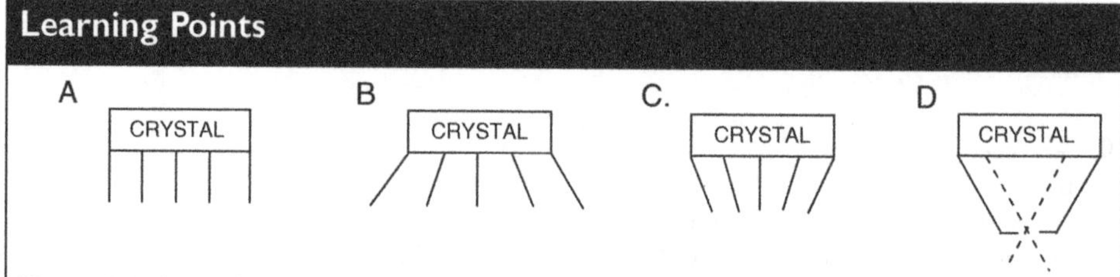

Figure 9.1 Collimators

Types of collimators:

A. **Parallel hole:** most commonly used with a 400mm camera. The field of view (FOV) and in air sensitivity are the same for all distances.
B. **Divergent hole:** A large FOV is obtained but the image minifies.
C. **Convergent hole:** A small FOV but the image magnifies.
D. **Pinhole:** Produces a magnified but inverted image.

15. A. True.
B. False: A divergent hole collimator does allow a large field of view to be obtained but it minifies the image.
C. False: A convergent hole collimator magnifies the image when a small field of view is obtained. This is used in imaging small organs or children.
D. True.
E. True: It is used in imaging superficial small organs such as the thyroid.

Sharp, Gemmell, & Murray. *Practical Nuclear Medicine*, 3rd edn, Springer, 2005. pp. 4–9.
Electronic Learning Database, E-Learning for Healthcare, Radiology—Integrated Training Initiative (R-ITI) – www.e-lfh.org.uk
Module: 8a_112: Image Formation with a Gamma Camera.

16. A. False: It is made of sodium iodide and activated with a trace of thallium.
B. False: It is one large crystal.
C. True.
D. True.
E. False: It is fragile, hygroscopic and easily damaged by temperature change.

Sharp, Gemmell, & Murray. *Practical Nuclear Medicine*, 3rd edn, Springer, 2005. pp. 4–9.

17. A. True.
B. True.
C. True.
D. True.
E. False: Photomultiplers are a key component in a gamma camera.

Powsner & Powsner. *Essential Nuclear Medicine Physics*, 2nd edn, Blackwell Publishing, 2006. pp. 65–84.

18. A. False: Collimator locates the radioactive source within the patient along its line of sight, without it no image would be formed.
B. True.
C. False: The spatial resolution from a CT scanner is far superior to that of a gamma camera.
D. True: The numbers of electrons are increased at each dynode, producing a cascade effect.
E. False: The main cause of variation in the image is electronic in nature.

Electronic Learning Database, E-Learning for Healthcare, Radiology—Integrated Training Initiative (R-ITI) – www.e-lfh.org.uk
Module: 8a_112: Image Formation with a Gamma Camera.

19. A. True: Resolution improves with a thinner crystal.
B. True: Spatial resolution improves with a smaller of the width of the holes in the collimator.
C. True: The longer the holes of the collimator, the better the spatial resolution.
D. False: Count rate affects the brightness of the pixel and not the spatial resolution if acquired over the same period of time.
E. False: The photomultiplier tubes acts as an amplifier and does not affect the spatial resolution.

Electronic Learning Database, E-Learning for Healthcare, Radiology—Integrated Training Initiative (R-ITI) – www.e-lfh.org.uk
Module: 8a_113: Image Quality.

20. A. False: Spatial resolution is assessed by imaging a line source, which gives the line spread function.
   B. False: Uniformity of field is assessed by using a flood field phantom.
   C. False: The typical system uniformity is approximately 2%.
   D. True: The intrinsic resolution of a gamma camera is the best resolution a camera can achieve.
   E. False: A cracked crystal appears as a defect in the image.

Electronic Learning Database, E-Learning for Healthcare, Radiology—Integrated Training Initiative (R-ITI) – www.e-lfh.org.uk
Module: 8a_118: Quality Assurance in Radionuclide Imaging.

21. A. True.
   B. True: You can have continuous or set and shoot acquisition.
   C. True.
   D. True.
   E. False: The counts per second per MBq received by a double- or triple-headed camera will be greater than that of a single-headed camera. Hence the system sensitivity will increase. The sensitivity of each individual head of the camera will not be affected.

Powsner & Powsner. *Essential Nuclear Medicine Physics*, 2nd edn, Blackwell Publishing, 2006. pp. 85–113.
Electronic Learning Database, E-Learning for Healthcare, Radiology—Integrated Training Initiative (R-ITI) – www.e-lfh.org.uk
Module: 8a_115: Single Photon Emission Computed Tomography.

22. A. True: It is corrected by a gamma attenuation algorithm when reconstructing the image.
   B. False: In SPECT, the spatial resolution is worse than in conventional gamma imaging but the contrast resolution is improved.
   C. True.
   D. False: Noise is increased in SPECT as the images are made up of fewer photons.
   E. False.

Powsner & Powsner. *Essential Nuclear Medicine Physics*, 2nd edn, Blackwell Publishing, 2006. pp. 85–113.

23. A. True.
   B. True.
   C. False: Overlying structures are resolved during 3D reconstruction.
   D. True.
   E. True: The views are reconstructed to slices which can be used to form a 3D image.

24. A. True.
   B. False: This will lead to an increase of the count of the image but the resolution is a factor of the system and not the patient.
   C. False: Resolution improves with a high resolution collimator.
   D. False.
   E. False.

Electronic Learning Database, E-Learning for Healthcare, Radiology—Integrated Training Initiative (R-ITI) – www.e-lfh.org.uk
Module: 8a_115: Single Photon Emission Computed Tomography.

25. A. False.
B. True.
C. False.
D. False.
E. True.

26. A. True.
B. True.
C. False: PET detects the gamma rays emitted as a result of annihilation between positrons and electrons.
D. False: PET imaging is based on detected two annihilation photons in coincidence.
E. True.

Powsner & Powsner. *Essential Nuclear Medicine Physics*, 2nd edn, Blackwell Publishing, 2006. pp. 114–27.
Electronic Learning Database, E-Learning for Healthcare, Radiology—Integrated Training Initiative (R-ITI) – www.e-lfh.org.uk
Module: 8a_116: Positron Emission Tomography (PET).

27. A. True.
B. True.
C. True.
D. True.
E. True.

28. A. True.
B. True.
C. True.
D. True.
E. True.

Powsner & Powsner. *Essential Nuclear Medicine Physics*, 2nd edn, Blackwell Publishing, 2006. pp. 37–64.

29. A. True.
B. True.
C. True.
D. False: Patient dose is of similar magnitude as that of SPECT.
E. True: ^{18}F has a half-life of 110 minutes whilst $^{99}Tc^{m}$ has a half-life of 6 hours.

30. A. False: The dose is dependent on the emitted energy of the gamma rays.
B. False: The dose is proportional to the administered radioactivity.
C. False: It is dependent on the biological half-life, physical half-life and the effective half-life.
D. False: The effective dose is measured in Sieverts.
E. False: The received dose is unaffected by the number of images acquired.

Dendy & Heaton. *Physics For Diagnostic Radiology*, 2nd dn, Institute of Physics Publishing, 1999. pp. 121–46.

31. A. True.
B. True.
C. False: The absorbed dose does not increase proportionally as decay is not a linear process.
D. False: The absorbed dose does not increase in proportion with an increase in the energy of gamma radiation.
E. False: Increasing the renal excretion rate decreases the biological half live hence it reduces the absorbed dose.

Electronic Learning Database, E-Learning for Healthcare, Radiology—Integrated Training Initiative (R-ITI) – www.e-lfh.org.uk
Module: 8a_045: Nuclear Medicine: Practical Radiation Protection of Patients.

32. A. True.
B. False: It is approximately 18mSv for a ^{201}Th heart scan.
C. True.
D. True.
E. True.

Dendy & Heaton. *Physics For Diagnostic Radiology*, 2nd dn, Institute of Physics Publishing, 1999. pp. 121–46.

33. A. False: Ideally should be a pure gamma emitter as beta radiation contributes to patient dose with no role in image formation.
B. False: Lead aprons are ineffective against high energy gamma rays.
C. True.
D. False: At such high energies, the contribution from photoelectric interactions is negligible.
E. False.

Electronic Learning Database, E-Learning for Healthcare, Radiology—Integrated Training Initiative (R-ITI) – www.e-lfh.org.uk
Module: 8a_117: Radiation Safety in Radionuclide Imaging.

34. A. True.
B. False: Only consultant radiologists with experience in nuclear medicine are considered to have sufficient experience to hold a licence. Hence they are the practitioner for all the nuclear medicine tests within their department.
C. True.
D. True.
E. False: Each licence is issued to individual clinicians for specified procedures at a particular hospital.

Notes for Guidance on the Clinical Administration of Radiopharmaceuticals and Use of Sealed Radioactive Sources—March 2006.
http://www.arsac.org.uk/notes_for_guidance/documents/ARSACNFG2006Corrected06-11-07.pdf.
Electronic Learning Database, E-Learning for Healthcare, Radiology—Integrated Training Initiative (R-ITI) – www.e-lfh.org.uk
Module: 8a_034: MARS and RSA.

35. A. True.
B. True: The applicant has to demonstrate that there is adequate numbers of trained staff within a well equipped nuclear medicine department.
C. True.
D. True.
E. True.

Notes for Guidance on the Clinical Administration of Radiopharmaceuticals and Use of Sealed Radioactive Sources—March 2006.
http://www.arsac.org.uk/notes_for_guidance/documents/ARSACNFG2006Corrected06-11-07.pdf
Electronic Learning Database, E-Learning for Healthcare, Radiology—Integrated Training Initiative (R-ITI) – www.e-lfh.org.uk
Module: 8a_034: MARS and RSA.

36. A. True.
B. True.
C. False: An active nuclear medicine department will have an excess of the exemption limits of radioactive substances hence registration is necessary.
D. False: Records of disposal are sent to the Environment Agency which is available for public viewing.
E. True.

Radioactive Substances Act 1993.
http://www.opsi.gov.uk/acts/acts1993/ukpga_19930012_en_1.

37. A. True.
B. True: The drain must be labelled for this purpose.
C. True.
D. True.
E. True.

Electronic Learning Database, E-Learning for Healthcare, Radiology—Integrated Training Initiative (R-ITI) – www.e-lfh.org.uk
Module: 8a_117: Radiation Safety in Radionuclide Imaging.
Module: 8a_046: Nuclear Medicine. Other Practical Radiation Protection Issues

38. A. True.
B. False: Patients containing radioactivity are a source of external radiation hence distance, shielding, and time should be applied to protect staff and the public.
C. True.
D. False: Lead aprons are not worn by nuclear medicine radiographers as it provides suboptimal protection.
E. True.

Sharp, Gemmell, & Murray. *Practical Nuclear Medicine*, 3rd edn, Springer, 2005. pp. 91–112.
Electronic Learning Database, E-Learning for Healthcare, Radiology—Integrated Training Initiative (R-ITI) – www.e-lfh.org.uk
Module: 8a_044: Nuclear Medicine: Practical Radiation Protection of Staff.

39. A. True: This will reduce the dose to the gonads and to the pelvic bone marrow in radionuclides which are excreted by the kidneys.

B. False: Children should receive less activity than adults and the administered activity is calculated according to the weight of the child.

C. True: ARSAC recommends such guidance in order to constrain foetal doses.

D. True: This may be performed based on risk assessment.

E. False: Breast-fed infants will be exposed to an internal radiation dose from the activity secreted in the breast milk in addition to the external radiation during close contact with their lactating mother.

Electronic Learning Database, E-Learning for Healthcare, Radiology—Integrated Training Initiative (R-ITI) – www.e-lfh.org.uk
Module: 8a_117: Radiation Safety in Radionuclide Imaging.

40. A. True.

B. False: There are no dose limits in medical exposures but all doses must be kept as low as reasonably practicable.

C. True.

D. False: Diagnostic reference levels are set by the Administration of Radioactive Substances Advisory Committee.

E. True.

chapter

10 ULTRASOUND

QUESTIONS

1. **Concerning diagnostic ultrasound:**

   A. The lower the transmitted frequency, the greater the depth that can be scanned.
   B. It has a wavelength in soft tissue of 0.1–1.5 nanometres.
   C. It is reflected from a surface between two media that have different acoustic impedances.
   D. The ultrasound beam cannot be focused.
   E. Ionization of soft tissue may occur at frequencies greater than 1MHz.

2. **The following statements are true for diagnostic ultrasound:**

   A. It uses frequencies between 2–15MHz.
   B. It is audible.
   C. It is a wave phenomenon.
   D. The speed of ultrasound remains constant through different tissue.
   E. It cannot travel through a vacuum.

3. **Concerning ultrasound:**

   A. It has an average speed of 300m/s in soft tissue.
   B. A change in acoustic impedance between two media causes refraction.
   C. The time gain compensator (TGC) can be used to decrease the amplitude of strong echoes behind fluid filled structures.
   D. TGC is used to enhance echoes from deeper structures.
   E. Using tissue harmonic imaging in the obese patient can improve tissue contrast as it suppresses the effect of sidelobe and reverberation artefacts.

4. **Regarding ultrasound:**

   A. Ultrasound is a transverse wave.
   B. The intensity of ultrasound is measured in watts per centimetre squared.
   C. In pulse-echo imaging the depth of an interface d = ct, where c is the velocity of sound, and t is the time of travel of the pulse.
   D. Ultrasound travels through a medium by waves of compression and rarefaction.
   E. Attenuation of ultrasound results in the heating of tissues.

5. The velocity of ultrasound in tissue is affected by the:

A. Frequency of ultrasound.
B. Wavelength of ultrasound.
C. Temperature.
D. Tissue compressibility.
E. Tissue density.

6. Concerning diagnostic ultrasound:

A. The magnitude of echoes is proportional to the sum of impedances of tissues.
B. The acoustic impedance of a tissue is directly proportional to its density.
C. At the soft tissue–air interface, over 99% of the energy is reflected.
D. The velocity of sound in tissue tends to increase with the density of the tissue.
E. The acoustic impedance of a tissue is constant within the diagnostic frequency range.

7. In order to detect tissue boundaries with pulsed ultrasound:

A. It is desirable that the incident beam strikes the tissue surfaces at right angles.
B. The acoustic impedance on each side of the boundary should be the same.
C. At least 5% of the incident beam must be reflected back to the transducer.
D. There must be a difference between the product of density and propagation velocity for the tissues on each side of the boundary.
E. The reflective surface must be stationary.

8. In diagnostic ultrasound:

A. The velocity of sound in the liver is twice the velocity in muscle.
B. The velocity of sound is dependent of the temperature.
C. The absorption of ultrasound in tissues is frequency dependent.
D. For a constant angle of incidence, the deviation of the refracted ultrasound beam will be greater at a soft tissue–bone interface than at a muscle–fluid interface.
E. The acoustic impedance of tissue is inversely proportional to its density.

9. In ultrasound:

A. A frequency of greater than 10MHz is normally used for an abdominal scan.
B. 40% of ultrasound is reflected from a bone and muscle interface.
C. Refraction is a cause of spatial artefacts.
D. A piezoelectric crystal resonates at the frequency at which the wavelength is equal to the thickness of the crystal.
E. The maximum pulse repetition frequency (PRF) is limited by the maximum depth to be sampled.

10. Concerning ultrasound:

A. Ultrasound is converted to thermal energy as it propagates through tissue.
B. Fluid absorbs ultrasound to a greater degree than soft tissue.
C. Increased beam frequency decreases tissue absorption.
D. High frequency ultrasound is less penetrative than low frequency ultrasound.
E. For a given beam frequency, lung attenuates more than blood.

11. Ultrasound transducer:

A. Ultrasound is generated and detected by thin piezoelectric discs, commonly made of lead zirconate titanate (PZT).
B. The transducer thickness is chosen to guarantee resonance at the required frequency.
C. A backing layer is included to ensure rapid damping of the transducer vibration.
D. An impedance matching layer is incorporated to achieve maximum energy transfer in and out of the patient.
E. The impedance matching layer results in a longer pulse and therefore has an adverse effect on pulse damping.

12. Regarding ultrasound:

A. The piezoelectric effect is when an electric potential is produced when a crystal undergoes a mechanical distortion.
B. The resonance frequency of the transducer crystal is dependent on the crystal diameter and not on its thickness.
C. Scatter in all directions occurs when the imaged structure has dimensions smaller than a wavelength of the ultrasound beam.
D. Scatter allows small structures to be visualized as some scatter will reach the transducer.
E. Aliasing is a pulsed Doppler artefact.

13. Regarding ultrasound:

A. High Quality (Q) transducers are more efficient transmitters.
B. Low Q transducers are more efficient receivers.
C. A heavily damped transducer has a low Q factor.
D. A lightly damped transducer has a high Q factor.
E. The thicker the piezoelectric crystal the higher the resonance frequency.

14. In ultrasound imaging:

A. dB is the unit of acoustic impedance.
B. Acoustic impedance is the product of density and frequency.
C. At the interface between tissues of similar acoustic impedance a large proportion of the beam is reflected.
D. Absorption of ultrasound in tissues results in heat production.
E. A mirror image artefact commonly occurs at the diaphragm.

15. Ultrasound:

A. Ultrasound travels faster in soft tissue than bone.
B. The average velocity of ultrasound in soft tissue is 1540 metres per second.
C. Acoustic impedance is measured in milligrams per metre per second.
D. A-mode scans can be used to measure the diameter of the eye.
E. Echoes from A-mode scans are displayed as a series of dots.

16. Regarding ultrasound:

A. Ultrasound is attenuated exponentially with depth.
B. Attenuation varies with frequency.
C. Attenuation of ultrasound is measured in kilograms per square metre per second.
D. Scatter contributes towards attenuation.
E. Cavitation is a resonance phenomenon.

17. Attenuation in ultrasound:

A. Consists of absorption, reflection, and scatter.
B. Attenuation decreases with increasing frequency.
C. Attenuation is halved when the path length is doubled.
D. Attenuation in bone is lower than attenuation in soft tissue.
E. Absorption is the conversion of sound to heat.

18. An ultrasound transducer:

A. Converts mechanical energy into ultrasound and vice versa.
B. Operates on the principal of the piezoelectric effect.
C. A continuous alternating voltage applied to a transducer produces pulsed ultrasound.
D. Frequency increases as the thickness of the transducer increases.
E. Frequency bandwidth increases with decreasing pulse length.

19. Regarding ultrasound beam characteristics:

A. The near field (Fresnel zone) diverges.
B. The far field (Fraunhofer zone) extends a distance proportional to the square of the diameter of the transducer.
C. Side lobes are caused by radial (non-thickness) mode vibration of the transducer disc.
D. Side lobes may cause image artefacts.
E. Increasing the frequency or the diameter of the transducer increases the length of the near zone and decreases the divergence of the far zone.

20. Concerning ultrasound:

A. Axial resolution is the ability of the ultrasound beam to separate two interfaces along the axis of the beam.
B. Azimuthal (lateral) resolution is the ability of ultrasound beam to separate two structures side by side at the same depth.
C. Axial resolution is generally better than lateral resolution.
D. In the axial plane, two interfaces will be differentiated if the distance between them is less than half of the spatial pulse length.
E. Resolution in the near field improves with focusing and a larger diameter transducer.

21. Lateral resolution:

A. It is equal to the beam diameter.
B. Increasing frequency improves lateral resolution for a given transducer diameter.
C. Lateral resolution does not vary with distance from the transducer.
D. A small transducer improves lateral resolution for any given distance.
E. Lateral resolution is determined by damping.

22. In ultrasound a phased array can vary:

A. The direction of beam.
B. The focal length.
C. The axial resolution.
D. The lateral resolution.
E. The pulse repetition frequency.

23. A-mode scans:

A. Amplitudes of echoes are presented as vertical deflections on the screen.
B. A-mode scans are inaccurate in measuring the amplitude of echoes.
C. The distance between targets cannot be measured with A-mode scans.
D. Dedicated A-mode equipment is still frequently used.
E. Can measure foetal biparietal diameter.

24. B-mode scans:

A. The beam axis (scan line) is swept through the area of interest to define a scan plane.
B. The echoes from all scan lines are displayed as a two dimensional image of the scan plane.
C. The amplitude of the echo is inversely proportional to the brightness of the corresponding point on the display.
D. Multiple pulses are required per line to build up a single image.
E. Can be used to produce a cross-sectional image of the eye and the orbit.

25. Time-gain compensation is used to:

A. Improve lateral resolution.
B. Compensate for the difference in time between the front and back of a signal.
C. Compensate for the difference in attenuation between different tissues.
D. Compensate for the effect of attenuation with distance travelled within a medium.
E. Obtain similar intensity signals from all similar boundaries.

26. M-mode scans:

A. Display the position of reflecting surfaces along a single scan line versus time.
B. The vertical co-ordinate represents time whilst the horizontal co-ordinate represents depth.
C. The echo brightness indicates the echo amplitude.
D. Each transmission-reception sequence is summated with the previous M-mode line.
E. Are primarily used in cardiac imaging.

27. Deep lying structures are most readily displayed ultrasonically by:

A. Increasing the frequency to improve the resolution detail.
B. Reducing the frequency to lessen the effect of absorption.
C. Increasing the brightness of the display to show the weaker echoes.
D. Increasing the ultrasound intensity.
E. Using an alternative direction of scan to avoid overlying reflecting structures.

28. In ultrasound:

A. Contrast agents improve image quality and information by increasing reflections from tissue containing the agents.
B. Microbubbles used as ultrasound contrast agents are between 1 and 10 micrometre in diameter.
C. Microbubbles can be destroyed by low intensity ultrasound.
D. Tissue harmonic imaging can increase reverberation artefacts.
E. Tissue harmonic imaging can decrease scatter and distortion from fatty tissues, and hence leads to an improvement in image contrast.

29. The Doppler effect:

A. Is a change in the frequency of the reflected ultrasound wave caused by reflector motion.
B. If the reflector is moving towards the source, the reflected frequency is lower than the incident frequency.
C. If the reflector is stationary to the source, the reflected frequency is equal to the incident frequency.
D. Measurement of Doppler shift frequency yields information about reflector motion.
E. The calculation of the change in frequency involves the sine of the angle between the incident and reflected direction.

30. Doppler shift frequency is directly proportional to:

A. The angle of the ultrasound (US) beam.
B. The speed of the target material.
C. The intensity of the US beam.
D. The size of the target material.
E. The frequency of the US beam.

31. Concerning pulsed Doppler ultrasound:

A. The maximum Doppler shift frequency that can be detected is half the PRF.
B. Depth assessment requires gating.
C. The change in frequency is greatest with the beam perpendicular to the direction of flow.
D. Sound velocity is increased by increased source motion.
E. The intensity of the back scattered signal is independent of the beam frequency.

32. Concerning the Doppler effect:

A. It produces a change in the velocity of sound reflected off a moving object.
B. A US beam parallel to the direction of movement gives the largest change in frequency.
C. It produces a change in frequency which is inversely proportional to the velocity of sound in the medium.
D. It causes an increase in frequency when the object is moving towards the transducer.
E. It requires a higher frequency than would be used for imaging.

33. Regarding Doppler ultrasound:

A. The Doppler shift frequency is equal to 1 over the transmitted frequency.
B. Velocity of blood flow is most accurately measured when the ultrasound beam is less than 60° to the direction of blood flow.
C. There is a maximum velocity which can be detected.
D. Spectral analysis of pulsed wave Doppler signals is usually accomplished using an autocorrelation technique.
E. PRF can be a limiting factor in the detection of signals from deep vessels.

34. Concerning pulsed Doppler US:

A. Doppler signals should preferably be acquired at angles between 30 and 60 degrees.
B. The Nyquist limit is determined by the PRF.
C. There is a maximum velocity that can de detected.
D. Typical Doppler shift frequencies produced diagnostically are inaudible.
E. Using high PRF avoids range ambiguity.

35. Regarding ultrasound:

A. Duplex scanning is a combination of Doppler measurement with a real time B-scan image.
B. Doppler shift frequency decreases through stenoses.
C. A lower PRF is required to visualize deeper vessels.
D. Power Doppler differentiates between areas with flow and areas devoid of flow.
E. Power Doppler is not subject to aliasing.

36. Biological effects of ultrasound:

A. Tissue heating occurs in the therapeutic range.
B. Acoustic streaming results from ultrasound energy being absorbed by a medium and has the potential to cause cellular damage.
C. Transient (unstable) cavitation occurs when changes in pressure cause microbubbles to expand and contract until they implode with high temperature rises causing profound cellular damage.
D. Transient cavitation most commonly occurs at low pressure and high frequencies.
E. If mechanical index (MI) reaches 0.25 there is a possibility of minor damage to neonatal lung or intestine and exposure time should be limited.

37. Intensity of diagnostic ultrasound:

A. The highest intensity that can be measured in an ultrasound beam is the spatial peak temporal average intensity (ISPTA).
B. The intensity of an ultrasound beam in water is greatest in the focal region.
C. The time-averaged intensity must never exceed $100mW/cm^2$.
D. ISPTA is generally highest in pulsed Doppler mode.
E. To estimate intensity in tissue, the acoustic pressure in water is measured using a hydrophone and a derating factor is applied to allow for the effects of attenuation.

38. In ultrasound:

A. The thermal index (TI) gives an indication of the temperature rise in tissue.
B. TI is the ratio of the in situ acoustic power to the power required to increase the tissue temperature by 10°C.
C. TIB refers to the thermal index to be used if bone is situated at the surface (i.e. transcranial applications).
D. The mechanical index (MI) is defined as the derated peak rarefactional pressure divided by the square root of frequency.
E. MI is a guide to the likelihood to cavitation.

39. Thermal index (TI) in ultrasound:

A. Is inversely proportional to the power emitted.
B. A TI of less than 0.5 is considered safe.
C. The scanning time of an embryo or foetus should be reduced when the thermal index is greater than 1.
D. Particular care should be taken to reduce output and minimize the exposure time of an embryo or foetus when scanning a febrile patient.
E. Real time values of TI and MI must always be displayed on the scanner.

40. Tissue heating in ultrasound:

A. Tissue heating damaging foetal dividing cells during the first 8 weeks of gestation is of particular concern.
B. Temperature increase to the foetus in excess of 1.5°C is potentially hazardous and exposure time should be limited.
C. B-mode causes a higher temperature rise than pulsed Doppler mode for the same given time.
D. The temperature rise in soft tissue is greater than bone.
E. Pre-existing temperature elevation and the heat from the probe are additives to tissue heating.

chapter

10 ULTRASOUND

ANSWERS

1. A. True.
   B. False: The wavelength in soft tissue is between 0.1–1.5 millimetres.
   C. True: The greater the difference in acoustic impedance, the greater the fraction reflected.
   D. False: It can be focused either by applying an acoustic lens to the transducer or by using curved transducer crystals. In array transducers focusing can also be achieved electronically.
   E. False: Only ionizing radiation, such as x-rays and gamma rays, can cause ionization in tissue. Ultrasound is a mechanical sound wave and therefore cannot cause this.

Allisy-Roberts & Williams. *Farr's Physics for Medical Imaging*, 2nd edn, Saunders Elsevier, 2008. pp. 149–150.

2. A. True.
   B. False: The upper limit of human hearing is 20KHz.
   C. True.
   D. False.
   E. True.

3. A. False: It has an average of 1540m/s in soft tissue.
   B. False: It is a change in the speed of sound which causes refraction.
   C. True.
   D. True: TGC applies more amplification to echoes from deeper depth hence compensating for the effect of attenuation.
   E. True.

Allisy-Roberts & Williams. *Farr's Physics for Medical Imaging*, 2nd edn, Saunders Elsevier, 2008. pp. 149–50.

4. A. False: Ultrasound is a longitudinal wave; the molecules vibrate back and forth in the same direction as the wave is travelling.
   B. True.
   C. False: This would actually give twice the depth as the pulse has travelled to the interface and returned in this time.
   D. True.
   E. True.

Kremkau. *Diagnostic Ultrasound—Principles and Instruments*, 7th edn, Saunders Elsevier, 2006. pp. 16–46.

5. A. False: The velocity is a constant for a given medium, a change in frequency will produce a corresponding change in wavelength.
B. False: As above.
C. True: The velocity of sound is temperature dependent because tissue density varies with tissue temperature.
D. True: $c = 1/\sqrt{K\rho}$ where K is compressibility and ρ is density. Therefore the greater the compressibility, the lower the velocity.
E. True: The greater the density, the lower the velocity.

Dendy & Heaton. *Physics for Diagnostic Radiology*, 2nd edn, IOP Publishing Ltd., 1999. p. 332.

6. A. False: The reflected intensity is related to the difference in impedance divided by the sum of impedances at an interface.
B. True.
C. True.
D. False: Velocity of sound is inversely proportional to the square root of the tissue density.
E. True: Acoustic impedance depends on the density and speed of sound, neither of which are frequency dependent.

Hennerici & Neuerburg-Heusler. 'Vascular diagnosis with ultrasound: Clinical reference with case studies', *Thieme*, p. 1

7. A. True.
B. False: Interfaces are detected when there is a difference in acoustic impedance.
C. False: Reflection coefficients for all soft tissue interfaces are less than 5%, for example the soft tissue—-muscle interface has a reflection coefficient of 0.04%.
D. True: Acoustic impedance = density × velocity.
E. False: Heart valves are seen despite not being stationary.

Kremkau. *Diagnostic Ultrasound—Principles and Instruments*, 7th edn, Saunders Elsevier, 2006. pp. 22–6.
Electronic Learning Database, E-Learning for Healthcare, Radiology—Integrated Training Initiative (R-ITI) – www.e-lfh.org.uk
Module: 8a_120: Ultrasound:the Pulse-Echo Principle.

8. A. False: There is minimal change in velocity within soft tissues hence an assumption of 1540m/s is used.
B. True: For example the velocity of sound in water at 20°C is 1480m/s but is 1570m/s at 37°C.
C. True: Absorption is a major component of the attenuation of ultrasound which is frequency dependent.
D. True: The greater the difference in speed of sound between two media, the greater the degree of refraction.
E. False.

Kremkau. *Diagnostic Ultrasound—Principles and Instruments*, 7th edn, Saunders Elsevier, 2006. pp. 27–44.

9. A. False: 3.5–5MHz is generally used for a general purpose scan of an adult abdomen.
B. True.
C. True.
D. False: The resonant frequency corresponds to a wavelength that is twice the thickness of the crystal.
E. True.

Allisy-Roberts & Williams. *Farr's Physics for Medical Imaging*, 2nd edn, Saunders Elsevier, 2008. pp. 147–68.
Electronic Learning Database, E-Learning for Healthcare, Radiology—Integrated Training Initiative (R-ITI) – www.e-lfh.org.uk
Module: 8a_121: Ultrasound: Generation, Detection, Focusing and Resolution.

10. A. True.
B. False: Fluid attenuates ultrasound less than soft tissue, hence post cystic enhancement.
C. False.
D. True.
E. True.

11. A. True.
B. True.
C. True.
D. True.
E. False: Impedance matching layers provide further damping in addition to achieving maximum energy transfer.

Kremkau. *Diagnostic Ultrasound—Principles and Instruments*, 7th edn, Saunders Elsevier, 2006. pp. 54–81.
Allisy-Roberts & Williams. *Farr's Physics for Medical Imaging*, 2nd edn, Saunders Elsevier, 2008. pp. 150–4.

12. A. True.
B. False: Resonance of the crystal is dependent on the thickness and not the diameter.
C. True.
D. True.
E. True.

13. A. True: Quality (Q) = Energy lost per cycle / energy stored per cycle. A good transmitter will lose more energy into the medium and therefore will have a high Q. Continuous wave transducers are examples of transducers with a high Q.
B. True: To receive echoes, however, the transducer must operate with a short pulse and therefore have a low Q.
C. True: Q = frequency / bandwidth. A heavily damped transducer has a short pulse length and hence a broad bandwidth so Q will be low.
D. True: A lightly damped transducer has a long pulse length and hence a narrow bandwidth so Q will be high.
E. False: A thicker crystal has a lower resonance frequency and a longer wavelength than a thinner crystal.

Kremkau. *Diagnostic Ultrasound—Principles and Instruments*, 7th edn, Saunders Elsevier, 2006. pp. 54–81.
Allisy-Roberts & Williams. *Farr's Physics for Medical Imaging*, 2nd edn, Saunders Elsevier, 2008. p. 150.

14. A. False: The decibel (dB) is a logarithmic unit used to compare one intensity with a reference intensity.
B. False: Acoustic impedance = density × velocity of sound
C. False.
D. True.
E. True.

Electronic Learning Database, E-Learning for Healthcare, Radiology—Integrated Training Initiative (R-ITI) – www.e-lfh.org.uk
Module: 8a_122: Reflection, Scatter and Absorption.

15. A. False.
B. True.
C. False: Kilogram per metre square per second.
D. True.
E. False: Echoes from A-mode are displayed as spikes and in B-mode are displayed as a series of dots.

16. A. True.
B. True: Attenuation increases with frequency.
C. False: It is measured in decibels per centimetre (dB cm^{-1}).
D. True: Attenuation is made up of absorption and scatter.
E. True.

Allisy-Roberts & Williams. *Farr's Physics for Medical Imaging*, 2nd edn, Saunders Elsevier, 2008. pp. 154–5.

17. A. True.
B. False: Attenuation increases with increasing frequency.
C. False: Attenuation doubles when the path length is doubled.
D. False: Attenuation in bone is higher than in soft tissue.
E. True.

18. A. False: It converts electrical energy into ultrasound and vice versa.
B. True.
C. False: A continuous alternating voltage applied to a transducer produces continuous ultrasound.
D. False: Frequency decreases as the thickness of the transducer increases.
E. True.

Kremkau. *Diagnostic Ultrasound—Principles and Instruments*, 7th edn, Saunders Elsevier, 2006. pp. 54–81.

19. A. False: The beam in the near field is parallel and the beam in the far field diverges.
B. False: It is the near field which has a length related to the square of the diameter.
C. True.
D. True.
E. True.

Szabo. *Diagnostic Ultrasound Imaging: Inside out*, Academic Press, 2004. pp. 154–63.

20. A. True.
B. True.
C. True.
D. False: The best axial resolution achievable is half of the spatial pulse length. Interfaces must be further apart to be resolvable.
E. False: Resolution in the near field improves with focusing and a smaller diameter transducer.

Szabo. *Diagnostic Ultrasound Imaging: Inside out*, Academic Press, 2004. pp. 154–63.
Allisy-Roberts & Williams. *Farr's Physics for Medical Imaging*, 2nd edn, Saunders Elsevier, 2008. pp. 161–2.

21. A. True.
B. True.
C. False: Lateral resolution depends on beam width and this varies with distance from transducer.
D. False: A small transducer only improves lateral resolution when it is near the transducer, the beam becomes more divergent in the far field.
E. False: Lateral resolution is determined by frequency, focusing, transducer diameter and distance from the transducer.

Allisy-Roberts & Williams. *Farr's Physics for Medical Imaging*, 2nd edn, Saunders Elsevier, 2008. pp. 161–2.

22. A. True: The beam can be steered by altering the delay times between the excitation pulses which activate the individual transducer elements.
B. True: Electronic focusing is also achieved through altering delay times.
C. True: Axial resolution depends on pulse length which can be altered by changing the transmit frequency.
D. True: Lateral resolution depends on beam focusing which is varied by altering delay lines.
E. True: The PRF is just how frequently ultrasound pulses are sent out and is determined by the depth of interest. This can be varied with a phased array in the same way as it is with any other transducer.

Allisy-Roberts & Williams. *Farr's Physics for Medical Imaging*, 2nd edn, Saunders Elsevier, 2008. pp. 157.

23. A. True.
B. False.
C. False: The time between the vertical deflections can be converted to distance if the velocity of sound is known.
D. False: Dedicated A-mode equipment is rarely manufactured but it is used as an additional feature on B-scan equipment.
E. True.

Allisy-Roberts & Williams. *Farr's Physics for Medical Imaging*, 2nd edn, Saunders Elsevier, 2008. p. 155.

24. A. True.
B. True.
C. False: The amplitude of the echo is proportional to the brightness of the corresponding point on the display.
D. False: Only a single pulse is required but multiple pulses may be used if, for example, multiple focal zones are being used.
E. True.

Allisy-Roberts & Williams. *Farr's Physics for Medical Imaging*, 2nd edn, Saunders Elsevier, 2008. p. 156.
Electronic Learning Database, E-Learning for Healthcare, Radiology—Integrated Training Initiative (R-ITI) – www.e-lfh.org.uk
Module: 8a_123: The B-Scanner.

25. A. False.
B. False.
C. True.
D. True.
E. True.

Allisy-Roberts & Williams. *Farr's Physics for Medical Imaging*, 2nd edn, Saunders Elsevier, 2008. p. 156.

26. A. True.
B. False: The vertical co-ordinate represents depth whilst the horizontal co-ordinate represents time.
C. True.
D. False: Each transmission–reception sequence results in a new M-mode line being displayed alongside the previous one, thereby allowing changes in echo position to be appreciated.
E. True.

Allisy-Roberts & Williams. *Farr's Physics for Medical Imaging*, 2nd edn, Saunders Elsevier, 2008. p. 157.

27. A. False: Frequency is reduced to increase penetration at the cost of poorer resolution.
B. True.
C. False: Increasing the brightness of the display will also increase the brightness of the noise, hence it will not improve signal to noise ratio.
D. True: Increasing intensity will increase echo amplitude at depth.
E. True.

28. A. True.
B. True.
C. False: Microbubbles are destroyed by ultrasound of high intensity.
D. False: Tissue harmonic imaging tends to decrease reverberation artefacts.
E. True.

Allisy-Roberts & Williams. *Farr's Physics for Medical Imaging*, 2nd edn, Saunders Elsevier, 2008. p. 159.
Electronic Learning Database, E-Learning for Healthcare, Radiology—Integrated Training Initiative (R-ITI) – www.e-lfh.org.uk
Module: 8b_015: Ultrasound Contrast Agents.
Forsberg, Goldberg, & Raichlen. *Ultrasound Contrast Agents*, 2nd edn, Informa Healthcare, 2001.

29. A. True.
B. False: When the reflector is moving towards the source, the reflected frequency is higher than the incident frequency.
C. True.
D. True.
E. False: It involves the cosine of the angle between these directions.

Kremkau. *Diagnostic Ultrasound—Principles and Instruments*, 7th edn, Saunders Elsevier, 2006. pp. 157–77.
Allisy-Roberts & Williams. *Farr's Physics for Medical Imaging*, 2nd edn, Saunders Elsevier, 2008. pp. 163–7.

30. A. False: It is directly proportional to the cosine of the angle of incidence.
B. False.
C. False.
D. False.
E. True.

Kremkau. *Diagnostic Ultrasound—Principles and Instruments*, 7th edn, Saunders Elsevier, 2006. pp. 157–77.

31. A. True.
B. True: Return echoes are gated so only the echoes coming from the region of interest are analysed.
C. False: The greatest change in frequency is when the beam is parallel to the direction of flow (i.e. $\theta = 0$, Cos 0 = 1).
D. False: Sound velocity is dependent on density and compressibility, not on how fast a source is moving.
E. False: Backscatter is highly frequency dependent.

Electronic Learning Database, E-Learning for Healthcare, Radiology—Integrated Training Initiative (R-ITI) – www.e-lfh.org.uk
Module: 8a_130: Pulsed Wave Doppler: Theory and Practical Implementation.

32. A. False: In the Doppler effect, it is the frequency which changes and not the velocity.
B. True: An ultrasound beam parallel to the direction of movement will give the largest shift as $\theta = 0$, cos 0 = 1.
C. True.
D. True.
E. False.

Kremkau. *Diagnostic Ultrasound—Principles and Instruments*, 7th edn, Saunders Elsevier, 2006. pp. 157–77.

33. A. False.
B. True: This is because the velocity is related to the cosine of the angle. At a 60-degree angle, a 5-degree error in angle measurement gives an error of 15% in the cosine of the angle. At an 80-degree angle, the same 5-degree error in angle measurement would give an error of 50% in the cosine of the angle, resulting in large errors in velocity estimation.
C. False: There is no limit to the velocity that can be detected using continuous wave Doppler, a limit only applies when using pulsed Doppler.
D. False. Fast Fourier transforms are usually used to acquire spectral data from the Pulsed Doppler signal. Autocorrelation is used in Colour Doppler.
E. True: Enough time must be allowed for echoes to return from deep structures before the next pulse can be sent out.

Allisy-Roberts & Williams. *Farr's Physics for Medical Imaging*, 2nd edn, Saunders Elsevier, 2008. pp. 163–7.

34. A. True.
B. True.
C. True.
D. False: Typical Doppler shift frequencies produced are within audible range hence the use of loudspeakers as a primary output device.
E. False: Using a high PRF may create range ambiguity as echoes generated from deeper structures will arrive at the transducer shortly after the next pulse is transmitted and will be misregistered as coming from superficial structures.

35. A. True.
B. False.
C. True: More time must be allowed for echoes from deep structures to return to the transducer and therefore the number of pulses per second (PRF) has to be decreased.
D. True.
E. True: With Power Doppler it is the amplitude of the signal that is portrayed and therefore it does not matter if calculated frequency shift is inaccurate.

36. A. True.
B. True.
C. True.
D. False: Transient cavitation will not occur until the pressure reaches a certain threshold, this threshold pressure is higher at higher frequencies.
E. False: The mechanical index (MI) has to be greater than 0.3 for the possibility of damage.

Kremkau. *Diagnostic Ultrasound—Principles and Instruments*, 7th edn, Saunders Elsevier, 2006. pp. 319–33.

37. A. False: ISPTA refers to the spatial peak temporal average intensity, i.e. the intensity is measured at the position in the sound beam where intensity is highest but averaged over the pulse repetition period. Both the ISPPA (spatial peak pulse average) and the ISPTP (spatial peak temporal peak) measurements will be higher.
B. True.
C. False: ISPTA of 100mW/cm^2 is used in the International Electrotechnical Commission (IEC) standards but refers to a threshold above which manufacturers must provide further information relating to machine outputs. The US Food and Drug Administration (FDA) do set a maximum value for ISPTA but this is much higher at 720mW/cm^2 in tissue for general applications.
D. True: In pulsed Doppler mode the beam is stationary so every pulse will contribute to the average intensity. In B-mode or colour mode the beam is swept making the temporal average intensity lower.
E. True: An attenuation rate of 0.3dB/cm/MHz is assumed to estimate the intensity in tissue.

Kremkau. *Diagnostic Ultrasound—Principles and Instruments*, 7th edn, Saunders Elsevier, 2006. pp. 319–33.

38. A. True.
B. True.
C. False: There are three thermal indices: TIS for soft tissue, TIB for when there is bone near the focal region of the transducer, and TIC where bone is at the surface. TIC is the appropriate index for transcranial applications.
D. True.
E. True.

Kremkau. *Diagnostic Ultrasound—Principles and Instruments*, 7th edn, Saunders Elsevier, 2006. pp. 319–33.

39. A. False.
B. True.
C. True: If TI > 0.7 then it is recommended that exposure times when scanning a foetus should be reduced. At TI = 0.7 exposure time should be less than 60 minutes. At TI =1 exposure time should be less than 30 minutes.
D. True.
E. False: Indices only need to be displayed if MI > 1 in B mode and TI > 0.4 in Doppler mode. However manufacturers frequently display both indices even at lower values.

Statement on the Safe Use, and Potential Hazards of Diagnostic Ultrasound Prepared by the Safety Group of the British Medical Ultrasound Society. BMUS 2007. http://www.bmus.org/about-ultrasund/au-safetystatement.asp.

40. A. True.
B. True.
C. False: Pulsed Doppler mode has greater heating potential due to the high pulse repetition frequencies and the pulse lengths used.
D. False: Bone is associated with the highest temperature rise secondary to its high absorption coefficient.
E. True.

Kremkau. *Diagnostic Ultrasound—Principles and Instruments*, 7th edn, Saunders Elsevier, 2006. pp. 319–33.

Learning Points

Table 10.1 Relationship between frequency and wavelength in soft tissue

Frequency (f) in MHz	Wavelength (λ) in mm
1	1.5
2	0.8
5	0.3
8	0.2
10	0.15
15	0.1

(Speed of sound c = 1540m/s; $\lambda = c/f$)

Table 10.2 Velocity of ultrasound in various materials

Material	Average velocity (c) m/s
Air	330
Soft tissue	1540
Bone	3200

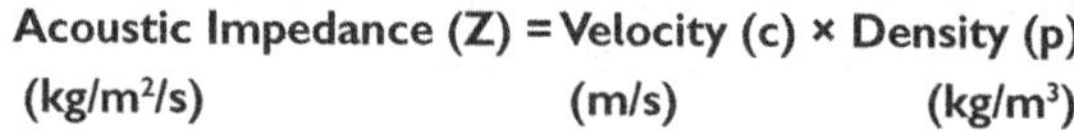

Acoustic Impedance (Z) = Velocity (c) × Density (p)
(kg/m²/s)
(m/s)
(kg/m³)

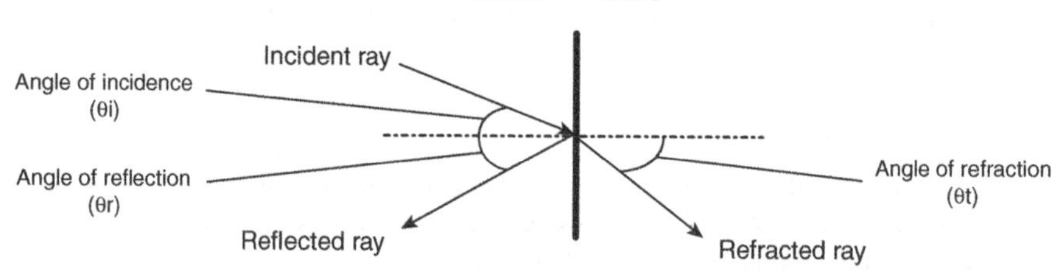

Law of reflection $\theta i = \theta r$

The angle of incidence (θi) equals the angle of reflection (θr).

Snell's Law of refraction $\frac{\sin \theta i}{\sin \theta t} = \frac{ci}{ct}$

Ratio of the sines of the incident and refraction angles is equal to the ratio of the sound velocities of the incidence (ci) and refraction (ct).

Figure 10.1 Reflection and refraction of the ultrasound beam

Law of reflection $\theta i = \theta r$

The angle of incidence (θi) equals the angle of reflection (θr).

Snell's Law of refraction $\frac{\sin \theta i}{\sin \theta t\ ct} = ci$

The ratio of the sines of the incident and refraction angles is equal to the ratio of the sound velocities of the incidence (ci) and refraction (ct).

Learning Points *(continued)*

Table 10.3 Reflection factors

Interface	Percentage of reflection (%)
Soft tissue—Gas	99.9
Muscle—Bone	30
Fat—Muscle	1
Blood—Muscle	0.1

Attenuation = Absorption + Scatter

Table 10.4 Tissue attenuation values at 1MHz

Material	Attenuation (dB cm^{-1})
Water	0.0022
Blood	0.18
Soft tissue	0.7
Bone	15
Lung	40

Beam characteristics

a = transducer radius, λ= wavelength of ultrasound

- Length of near field = a^2/λ

  ↑ radius → ↑ length
  ↓ radius → ↓ length
  ↑ wavelength (↓ frequency)→ ↓ length
  ↓ wavelength (↑ frequency)→ ↑ length

- Far field divergence $\sin\theta = 0.61\lambda/a$

  ↑ radius → ↓ $\sin\theta$ (↓ θ)
  ↓radius → ↑ $\sin\theta$ (↑ θ)
  ↑ wavelength (↓ frequency)→ ↑ $\sin\theta$ (↑ θ)
  ↓ wavelength (↑ frequency)→ ↓ $\sin\theta$ (↓ θ)

Learning Points *(continued)*

Doppler shift frequency (f_d) = $f_t - f_r = 2 f_t v \cos\theta / c$

T = Transducer
f_t = Transmitted frequency
f_r = Received frequency
v = Velocity of reflector
c = Speed of sound in medium
θ = Angle between the beam and moving object

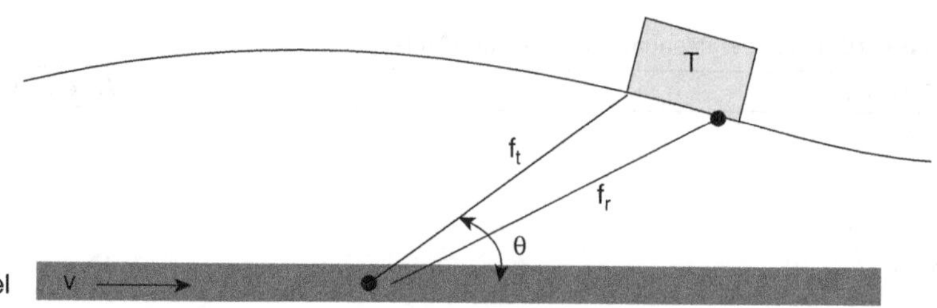

Figure 10.2 Doppler shift

Minimizing hazards in ultrasound:

- Keep power output as low as possible by increasing the overall gain.
- Keep exposure time to a minimum—e.g. probe should not be stationary for more than a few seconds; remove the probe when not examining the patient.
- Avoid scans when there is no medical justification.
- Involve medical physicist in risk assessing all ultrasound machines.
- Avoid pulse Doppler in early pregnancy or in the foetal or neonatal skull or spine.

chapter

11

MAGNETIC RESONANCE IMAGING

QUESTIONS

1. Regarding magnetic resonance imaging (MRI), the following statements are true:

A. The gyromagnetic ratio of a hydrogen (^{1}H) atom is 42.57MHzT^{-1}.
B. Spin-lattice relaxation describes the decay of transverse magnetization.
C. The time constant of T2 is always shorter than the time constant of T1 for the same tissue.
D. The Larmor frequency is defined as the sum of magnetic field strength and the gyromagnetic ratio.
E. Only hydrogen nuclei are said to be MR active.

2. Regarding MRI:

A. Faraday's law of induction states that the change in magnetic flux through a closed circuit induces an electromotive force (electric current) in the circuit.
B. The strength of the magnetic field (B) is measured in gauss (G).
C. The strength of the magnetic field (B) is measured in Tesla (T).
D. An MR active nucleus spins at its own precessional frequency.
E. The temperature of the sample does not affect the magnetic moments of hydrogen atoms.

3. In MRI, when resonance is induced by applying a radiofrequency pulse 90 degrees to the magnetic field (B_0), the following occurs:

A. The magnetic moments of the nuclei move out of phase of each other.
B. There is energy absorption.
C. Nuclei are flipped onto their sides in the transverse plane.
D. Some nuclei gain enough energy to join the high energy population.
E. The net magnetization vector rotates around the transverse plane inducing signal across the receiver coil by inducing a voltage within it.

4. Regarding MRI:

A. T1 recovery is due to interactions of intrinsic magnetic fields of adjacent nuclei.
B. T2 decay is due to dephasing caused by inhomogeneities of the external magnetic field.
C. Shim coils are used to combat inhomogeneities caused by the external magnetic field.
D. Water has high molecular motion (inherent energy) and therefore decays faster than fat.
E. Fat has low molecular motion (inherent energy) and therefore recovers quicker than water.

5. **Regarding MRI:**
   A. T1 recovery time is defined as the time it takes for 100% of the longitudinal magnetization to recover.
   B. Using a long TR (time to repetition) allows saturation to occur which enhances contrast.
   C. Fat has a short T1 recovery time.
   D. Water has a short T1 recovery time.
   E. In a proton density (PD) image, long TR is used to allow for saturation to occur to enhance contrast.

6. **Regarding MRI:**
   A. T2 decay of fat is shorter than that of water.
   B. T1 recovery of fat is shorter than that of water.
   C. T2 decay time is defined as the time it takes for 63% of transverse magnetization to be lost due to dephasing.
   D. T1 recovery time is defined as the time it takes for 63% of the longitudinal magnetization to recover.
   E. Tissues with low proton density such as air always appear as a low signal on an MR image.

7. **Regarding T1-weighted images:**
   A. Fat appears as a high signal.
   B. Slow flowing blood appears as a low signal.
   C. Water appears as a low signal.
   D. Typical time to echo (TE) is 70ms.
   E. Typical TR is 300–600ms.

8. **Regarding T2-weighted images using spin echo:**
   A. Cerebrospinal fluid (CSF) appears as high signal.
   B. Haemangiomas appear as high signal.
   C. Lipomas appear as high signal.
   D. Most pathologies are high signal on T2-weighted image.
   E. Typical TR is 2000ms.

9. **Regarding proton density(PD)-images:**
   A. Cortical bone appears as a high signal.
   B. CSF appears as a high signal.
   C. T1 effect is reduced by selecting short TE.
   D. T2 effect is reduced by selecting long TR.
   E. Typically uses short TE and long TR.

10. **Typical relaxation times of tissues in a field of 1T:**
   A. T2 of fat is typically 80ms.
   B. T1 of CSF is typically 150ms.
   C. T1 of water is typically 3000ms.
   D. T2 of CSF is typically 150ms.
   E. T2 of water is typically 3000ms.

11. The following are contraindications in MRI examinations:

A. Prosthetic heart valves.
B. Cochlear implants.
C. Cardiac pacemakers.
D. Intra-ocular ferrous foreign body.
E. Orthopaedic implants.

12. Regarding pulse sequences:

A. Spin echo uses a gradient to rephase spins.
B. Gradient echo uses a fixed flip angle of 90 degrees.
C. Gradient echo is a fast sequence when compared with spin echo.
D. Inhomogeneity effects of external magnetic fields are eliminated in spin echo sequences.
E. Gradient echo produces true T2 weighted images.

13. Regarding spin echo sequences:

A. In conventional spin echo sequences, a 180 degrees radio frequency (RF) pulse is used to rephase spins.
B. In fast or turbo spin echo sequences, TR is shorter than in conventional spin echo.
C. In T2 weighted scans on fast or turbo spin echo sequences, fat appears as high signal.
D. In T2 weighted scans on fast or turbo spin echo sequences, water appears as high signal.
E. In inversion recovery, the sequence starts with a 180 degree inverting pulse.

14. Regarding inversion recovery sequences:

A. The TR is the time between successive 180 degrees inverting pulse.
B. Time to inversion (TI) is the time between successive 180 degrees pulse.
C. Time to inversion (TI) is used as a T1 contrast control.
D. Fluid-attenuated inversion recovery (FLAIR) uses a short time to inversion (TI).
E. FLAIR is used to null the signal from CSF.

15. Regarding gradient echo sequences:

A. TR used in gradient echo is shorter than in spin echo.
B. As in spin echo, TR controls T1 weighting.
C. Moving blood appears as a low signal.
D. T1 image uses a large flip angle (60–120 degrees).
E. PD image uses a large flip angle (60–120 degrees).

16. Regarding slice selection:

A. The Z gradient selects axial slices.
B. Transmit bandwidth determines the slice thickness.
C. The steeper the slice select gradient, the thicker the slice.
D. Increasing transmit bandwidth increases axial spatial resolution.
E. The slice select gradient is also switched on during the 180 degrees pulse in spin echo sequences.

17. Regarding spatial encoding:

A. Phase encoding occurs during the 180 degrees rephasing pulse.
B. The slope of the phase encoding gradient determines spatial resolution.
C. In standard orientation, the phase encoding gradient produces a gradient across the x-axis.
D. In standard orientation, the frequency encoding gradient produces a gradient across the y-axis.
E. Frequency encoding is applied during TE.

18. The followings are true of signal to noise ratio (SNR) in MRI:

A. It increases with increasing field strength.
B. It is not related to the positioning of the receiver coils.
C. Increasing TE improves SNR.
D. Reducing the receiver bandwidth increases SNR.
E. It depends on flip angle.

19. The following are true of signal to noise ratio (SNR) in MRI:

A. Increasing TR increases signal.
B. Using a contrast medium increases signal to noise ratio (SNR).
C. By halving x,y FOV (field of view) (keeping slice thickness the same), the SNR is halved.
D. Increasing the number of signal averages (NSA/NEX), increases SNR.
E. Decreasing matrix size increases SNR.

20. Regarding spatial resolution in MRI:

A. Increasing FOV increases spatial resolution.
B. Increasing matrix size increases spatial resolution.
C. Increasing slice thickness decreases spatial resolution.
D. It is affected by the number of frequency encoding steps.
E. It is improved by using small coils.

21. Scan time depends on:

A. TR.
B. TE.
C. The number of frequency encoding steps.
D. The number of signal averages (NSA/NEX).
E. The number of slice encodings.

22. Regarding MRI:

A. Spatial encoding gradients are used to control FOV.
B. Slice selection gradient is used to control thickness.
C. The steeper the frequency, and phase encoding gradients, the larger the FOV.
D. In the frequency encoding direction, all information is acquired during TE.
E. In the phase encoding direction, all information is acquired after a single gradient step.

23. Regarding chemical shift artefact:

A. It occurs in the frequency encoding direction.
B. It can be remedied by using a stronger magnetic field.
C. It is decreased by decreasing receiving bandwidth.
D. It manifests as signal enhancement between areas of fat and water.
E. It can be combated by using short tau inversion recovery (STIR) sequences.

24. Regarding chemical shift artefact:

A. Reducing the FOV can be used to reduce chemical shift artefact.
B. It can be reduced by applying a reduced encoding gradient.
C. It is seen around the kidneys.
D. The Dixon technique is used to reduce its effect.
E. It can be seen in fat around the optic nerve.

25. Regarding artefacts:

A. Motion artefact occurs along the phase encoding direction.
B. Magnetic susceptibility artefacts are likely to be more noticeable in gradient echo (GRE) than on spin echo (SE) images.
C. Aliasing often occurs as a result of the FOV being too large.
D. Aliasing produces a wrap around image in the frequency encoding direction.
E. Chemical shift artefact occurs in the phase encoding direction.

26. Regarding contrast media used in MRI:

A. Gd-DTPA is a paramagnetic contrast agent.
B. Gd-DTPA shortens only T1 recovery time.
C. Gadolinium cannot be excreted by the body.
D. Gd-DTPA is contraindicated in pregnancy.
E. Gd-DTPA is contraindicated in sickle cell anaemia.

27. Regarding the use of contrast media in MRI:

A. Iron oxide (Fe_3O_4) is a positive contrast agent.
B. Area of uptake in normal tissue of iron oxide (Fe_3O_4) appears as a low signal.
C. Dysprosium-DTPA is known as a superparamagnetic contrast agent.
D. Iron oxide (Fe_3O_4) is known as a T1 enhancing agent.
E. Iron (Fe^{2+}) with four unpaired electrons can be used as paramagnetic contrast.

28. Regarding MRI safety:

A. Anyone with a cardiac pacemaker should be excluded from areas where stray fields are greater than 0.5mT.
B. A controlled area is defined as an area where stray fields are greater than 0.2T.
C. Static magnetic fields used can cause peripheral nerve stimulation.
D. Anaesthetized patients do not require hearing protection.
E. It is not recommended for pregnant patients to be scanned during the first three months of pregnancy.

29. Regarding the specific absorption ratio (SAR):

A. It is greater for large body parts.
B. It is greater for SE than for GRE.
C. It is greater for higher static fields.
D. It is greater for a 180 degree pulse than a 90 degree pulse.
E. Restricting whole body SAR to $1 Wkg^{-1}$ restricts whole body temperature rise to 0.5 degrees.

30. Regarding emergencies in MR environment:

A. Quenching superconducting electromagnets only results in minimal downtime.
B. Quenching does not result in damage to the superconducting magnet.
C. When quenching occurs, the room should be shut and ventilation turned off.
D. In the event of cardiac arrest in a superconducting magnet, the patient should remain in the MRI scanner with the arrest teams called in.
E. In case of fire, fire extinguishers can be used safely as normal.

31. Regarding electromagnets used in MRI:

A. Resistive magnets can be turned off instantaneously.
B. Permanent magnets can produce magnetic field up to 1.5T.
C. Permanent magnets typically weigh up to 80 tonnes.
D. Superconducting magnets are supercooled to absolute zero so that negligible resistance can be achieved.
E. A Faraday cage is used to eliminate fringe fields

32. Regarding MRI:

A. Shim coils are used to minimize magnetic field inhomogeneities.
B. For imaging purposes, homogeneity in the order of 30 parts per million (ppm) is required.
C. For spectroscopy, more homogenous an environment is required than for standard imaging.
D. Small stray fields are present in resistive magnets compared with superconductive electromagnets.
E. Insignificant stray fields are present in superconductive electromagnets.

33. Regarding the use of coils in MRI:

A. It is the switching off of shim coils that makes a loud banging noise.
B. The RF coils are positioned close to the patient in order to maximize the signal.
C. The RF coils produce a magnetic field at right angles to the main field.
D. The slice select (z-axis gradient) is switched on during the application of the RF pulse.
E. Surface coils are part of the main scanner.

34. Regarding safety in MRI:

A. Staff should not be exposed to more than 1T of static magnetic field to their whole body.
B. Staff should not be exposed to more than 5T of static magnetic field to their limbs.
C. Fringe fields depend on magnetic field strength.
D. The fringe field is independent of shielding.
E. A field strength of 3mT (30 Gauss) is chosen for the inner MR controlled area to avoid the projectile hazard.

35. Regarding safety in MRI:

A. There is a theoretical risk of peripheral nerve stimulation.
B. There is a theoretical risk of ventricular fibrillation.
C. For whole-body exposures, no adverse health effects are expected if the increase in body core temperature does not exceed 1°C.
D. In the case of infants and persons with cardiovascular impairment, the temperature increase should not exceed 0.5°C.
E. Burns are the most often reported MRI adverse incident in England.

36. The following are important considerations in quality assurance:

A. Uniformity.
B. Ghosting.
C. Geometric distortion.
D. Spatial resolution.
E. Slice thickness.

37. Regarding MR angiography (MRA):

A. 'Moving blood' appears as a high signal on an SE sequence.
B. Gradient echo sequences produce a high signal in blood.
C. Time of flight angiography uses a gradient echo sequence with a very short TR.
D. In phase-contrast MRA, the gradient strength may be adjusted to make the sequence sensitive to slow or fast flows.
E. Tissues with short T1 such as fat will always appear dark on time of flight (ToF) angiography.

38. In magnetic resonance imaging:

A. A STIR sequence is used to suppress a high signal such as that from fat.
B. Diffusion-weighted imaging utilizes the restriction of Brownian motion of water molecules to give a signal.
C. A diffusion-weighted imaging sequence on its own is normally sufficient for the interpretation of restricted water diffusion.
D. FLAIR is used to null a signal from fat.
E. Intracellular methaemoglobin appears as a high signal on T1-weighted image.

39. In magnetic resonance imaging:

A. Gadolinium-DTPA is normally used with a STIR sequence.
B. A fat saturation sequence uses an RF pulse centred on resonance frequency.
C. A fat saturation sequence requires a homogenous field.
D. STIR is usually combined with a fast spin echo.
E. Melanin appears as a high signal on T2.

40. Regarding MRI:

A. Superparamagnetic iron oxides are known to cause back pain.
B. Gd-DTPA has been reported to cause nephrogenic systemic fibrosis.
C. A water-suppressed STIR sequence is used in silicone breast imaging.
D. Manganese chelates are taken up by normal tissue and excreted in bile.
E. Functional MRI sequences are normally acquired using the ultrafast echo planar (GE-EPI) sequence.

chapter
11

MAGNETIC RESONANCE IMAGING

ANSWERS

1. A. True.
   B. False: This is spin–spin relaxation.
   C. True. The exception is pure water where T1 = T2.
   D. False: The Larmor frequency is defined as the product of magnetic field strength and the gyromagnetic ratio.
   E. False: Nuclei with an odd number of protons are said to be MR active. These include Hydrogen-1, Carbon-13, Fluorine-19, Phosphorous-31, Nitrogen-15, Oxygen-17, Sodium-23, etc.

Allisy-Roberts & Williams. *Farr's Physics for Medical Imaging*, 2nd edn, Saunders Elsevier, 2008. pp. 169–95.
Electronic Learning Database, E-Learning for Healthcare, Radiology—Integrated Training Initiative (R-ITI) – www.e-lfh.org.uk
Module: 8a_140: Introduction to MRI.

2. A. True: This electromagnetic induction is a basic principle of MRI. This principle is also applied to various other devices such as graphics tablets, loudspeakers, and electric guitar pickups.
   B. True.
   C. True: The strength of the magnetic field (B) is measured in both Gauss and Tesla. Tesla is the SI unit for magnetic flux density.
   D. False: They only precess when under the influence of an external magnetic field.
   E. False: The temperature is an important factor in determining whether a nucleus is in the high or low energy population, although in clinical imaging we often discount this as we assume that our patients are more or less the same temperature.

Westbrook. *MRI at a Glance*, Blackwell Science, 2002. pp. 12–13.

3. A. False: The magnetic moments of the nuclei move into phase with each other.
   B. True: The absorption of the radiofrequency (RF) energy at 90 degrees to B_0 causes an increased number of high energy spin-up nuclei.
   C. False: Nuclei are not physically flipped onto their sides, only the magnetic moments or the net magnetization vector moves.
   D. True: see B.
   E. True: This is the basis of signal detection.

Westbrook. *MRI at a Glance*, Blackwell Science, 2002. pp. 18–19.
Edelman, Hesselink, Zlatkin, & Crues. *Clinical Magnetic Resonance Imaging*, 3rd edn, Saunders Elsevier, 2005. p. 30.

4. A. False: it is due to spin-lattice energy transfer not spin–spin energy transfer as described in the question.
B. False: this is T2*. T2 dephasing is caused by spin–spin energy transfer.
C. True.
D. False: Water decays slower than fat because it has faster molecular motion (inherent energy) than fat. The faster the molecular motion the more difficult it is for a substance to release energy to its surroundings.
E. True: See D. T1 is short for fat.

Westbrook. *MRI at a Glance*, Blackwell Science, 2002. pp. 22–3.

5. A. False: T1 is defined as the time it takes for 63% of the longitudinal magnetization to recover.
B. False: Saturation occurs when there is a contrast difference between fat and water due to a difference in T1 recovery using short TRs.
C. True. Fat is able to absorb energy quickly so the T1 recovery time is short (i.e. their nuclei dispose of their energy to the surrounding fat tissue and return to B_0 in a short time).
D. False: Water has a long T1 recovery time because nuclei take a lot longer to dispose of their energy to the surrounding water tissue.
E. False: In PD weighted images, a long TR is used to allow full recovery of the longitudinal components of fat and water. There is no contrast difference and any differences seen are inherent to the proton density differences of each tissue. No saturation occurs.

Edelman, Hesselink, Zlatkin, & Crues. *Clinical Magnetic Resonance Imaging*, 3rd edn, Saunders Elsevier, 2005. p. 30–5.

6. A. True: Fat has a short T1 recovery and T2 decay compared to water.
B. True.
C. True: Or 37% remains.
D. True.
E. True.

Edelman, Hesselink, Zlatkin, & Crues. *Clinical Magnetic Resonance Imaging*, 3rd edn, Saunders Elsevier, 2005. pp. 30–5.
Table 11.1 illustrates different recovery and decay percentages at different time constants for T1 and T2.

Table 11.1 Different recovery and decay percentages for T1 and T2

Time Constants for T1	0	T1	2T1	3T1
Recovery (%)	0	63	86	95
Time Constants for T2	0	T2	2T2	3T2
Signal (%)	100	37	14	5

7. A. True.
B. False: Slow flowing blood appears as a high signal.
C. True: Water molecules do not recover much of their longitudinal magnetization during the short TR used in T1-weighted image.
D. False: Typically this is 10–30ms, although it is shorter in gradient echo sequences.
E. True: It is shorter in gradient echo sequences.

Westbrook. *MRI at a Glance*, Blackwell Science, 2002. p. 25.

8. A. True.
B. True.
C. False: Lipomas consist mostly of fat and therefore appear as a low signal because they lose most of their transverse coherence during a long TE. However, using fast spin echo (FSE), fat remains a high signal secondary to the J-coupling phenomenon.
D. True: Most pathologies have an increased water content and therefore appear as a high signal on T2 weighted images.
E. True.

Westbrook. *MRI at a Glance*, Blackwell Science, 2002. p. 26.

Learning Points

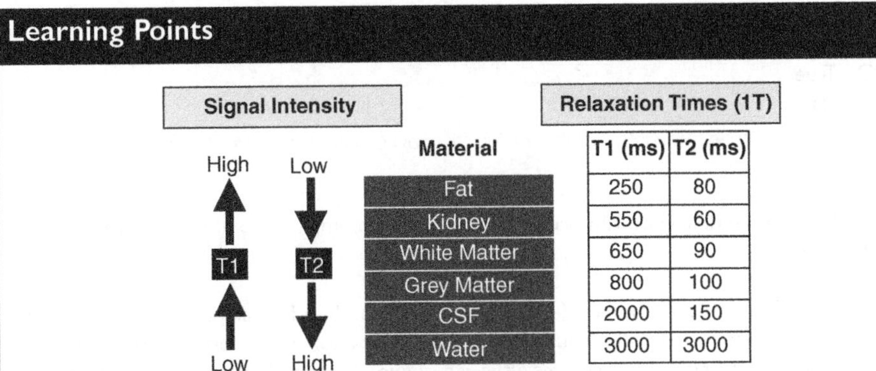

T1 (ms)	T2 (ms)
250	80
550	60
650	90
800	100
2000	150
3000	3000

Figure 11.1 Signal intensity versus relaxation times

Figures 11.1 and 11.2 illustrate the signal intensities and T1/T2 relaxation times in a field of 1 Tesla of different tissues.

For example, fat will have a high signal on T1 whereas water will have a high signal on T2. Typical relaxation times are displayed on the right in Figure 11.1 for different types of tissues. Note that fat may sometimes be quoted as high signal on T2 on FSE sequences and this is due to the J-coupling effect (see Q/A 13).

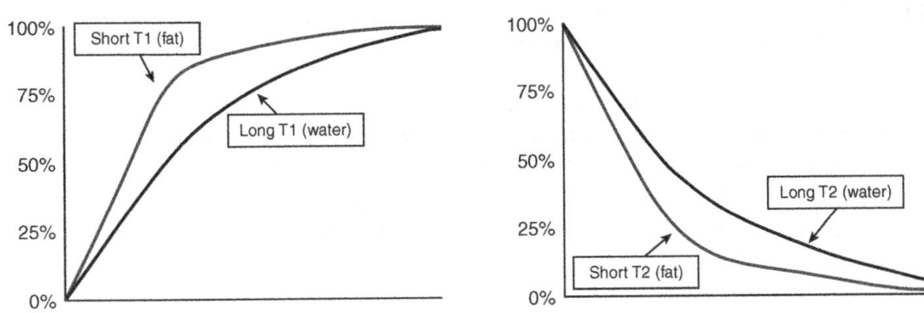

Figure 11.2 T1 and T2 differences between fat and water

T1 differences between fat and water

T2 differences between fat and water

Remember:

Fat = **F**astest

Fat signal recovers Faster than water (T1)
Fat signal decays Faster than water (T2)

9. A. False: Cortical bone always appears as a low signal on MR images regardless of the weighting as they have a low proton density and are effectively immobilized and therefore return little signal.
B. True.
C. False: T1 effect is reduced by selecting long TR.
D. False: T2 effect is reduced by selecting short TE.
E. True.

Westbrook. *MRI at a Glance*, Blackwell Science, 2002. p. 27.

10. A. True.
B. False: This is typically 2000ms (refer to Table 11.1).
C. True.
D. True.
E. True.

Allisy-Roberts & Williams. *Farr's Physics for Medical Imaging*, 2nd edn, Saunders Elsevier, 2008. p. 173.

11. A. False. Some deflection can occur but it is minimal compared to normal cardiac motion.
B. True.
C. True.
D. True. This is not uncommon (e.g. shrapnel injuries). Therefore all patients with suspected eye injuries are normally required to have a skull radiograph before MR examination. This is practised in most centres although opinion is divided regarding the potential risk of damage from intra-ocular foreign bodies.
E. False. Most orthopaedic implants show no deflection within the main magnetic fields. Although some theoretical risk of heating can occur secondary to induced currents, this is thought to be minimal.

Electronic Learning Database, E-Learning for Healthcare, Radiology—Integrated Training Initiative (R-ITI) – www.e-lfh.org.uk
Module: 8a_144: Metal and MR Safety.

12. A. False: Spin echo uses 180 degree RF pulse to rephase spins.
B. False: Gradient echo uses variable flip angles.
C. True.
D. True: It provides a true T2 weighting.
E. False: Because the gradient echo sequence does not completely eliminate the effect of inhomogeneities, it produces T2* images.

Westbrook. *MRI at a Glance*, Blackwell Science, 2002. pp.28–47.
Electronic Learning Database, E-Learning for Healthcare, Radiology—Integrated Training Initiative (R-ITI) – www.e-lfh.org.uk
Module: 8a_143: Basic Sequences.
Bitar, Leung, Perng, Tadros, Moody, Sarrazin, McGregor, Christakis, Symons, Nelson, & Roberts. 'MR pulse sequences: what every radiologist wants to know but is afraid to ask', *Radiographics*, 2006.

13. A. True.
B. False: Multiple TEs are used for a single TR and TR is longer than in conventional spin echo.
C. True. This is due to a succession of 180 degree RF pulses which reduce the spin–spin interactions in fat thereby increasing its T2 decay time (also known as J coupling).
D. True.
E. True.

See the Learning Point above and Figures 11.1 and 11.2.

Westbrook. *MRI at a Glance*, Blackwell Science, 2002. p.32.
Electronic Learning Database, E-Learning for Healthcare, Radiology—Integrated Training Initiative (R-ITI) – www.e-lfh.org.uk
Module: 8a_143: Basic Sequences.

14. A. True.
B. False: TI is the time between 180 degrees pulse and the 90 degree pulse.
C. True.
D. False. FLAIR uses long TIs, typically 1700–2200ms.
E. True.

Westbrook. *MRI at a Glance*, Blackwell Science, 2002. p.34.
Bitar, Leung, Perng, Tadros, Moody, Sarrazin, McGregor, Christakis, Symons, Nelson, & Roberts. 'MR pulse sequences: what every radiologist wants to know but is afraid to ask', *Radiographics*, 2006.

15. A. True.
B. True.
C. False. Moving blood appears as a high signal on a GRE sequence.
D. True.
E. False: It uses a small flip angle, typically between 5–20 degrees.

Westbrook. *MRI at a Glance*, Blackwell Science, 2002. pp.36–9.

16. A. True.
B. True.
C. False: The opposite is true.
D. False: Increasing transmit bandwidth increases slice thickness, thereby decreasing axial spatial resolution.
E. True: This is so that rephasing can be delivered specifically to the selected slice.

Westbrook. *MRI at a Glance*, Blackwell Science, 2002. pp.50–1.
Electronic Learning Database, E-Learning for Healthcare, Radiology—Integrated Training Initiative (R-ITI) – www.e-lfh.org.uk
Module: 8a_147: Localising the MRI Signal and Image Formation.

17. A. False: Phase encoding occurs before 180 degrees rephasing pulse.
B. True: Steeper gradients produce greater phase shifts between 2 points and increase the phase matrix FOV, thus improving spatial resolution along the phase axis.
C. False: Across the y-axis.
D. False: Across the x-axis.
E. True.

Westbrook. *MRI at a Glance*, Blackwell Science, 2002. pp.52–3.
Edelman, Hesselink, Zlatkin, & Crues. *Clinical Magnetic Resonance Imaging*, 3rd edn, Saunders Elsevier, 2005. pp. 39–42.

18. A. True.

B. False: The position of the receiver coil is important—it must be placed in the transverse plane perpendicular to the magnetic field.

C. False: Increasing TE reduces the SNR as more transverse magnetization dephases with time.

D. True: Reducing receiver bandwidth reduces the proportion of noise sampled relative to the signal, therefore boosting SNR (see Figure 11.3).

E. True: With a large flip angle, all available longitudinal magnetisation is converted into transverse magnetisation so that maximum signal is detected.

Westbrook. *Handbook of MRI Technique*, 3rd edn, Wiley-Blackwell, 2006. pp. 15–22.
Edelman, Hesselink, Zlatkin, & Crues. *Clinical Magnetic Resonance Imaging*, 3rd edn, Saunders Elsevier, 2005. pp. 90–6.

Learning Points

Encoding steps in a single Time to Repetition (TR)

Table 11.2 The basic differences between spin and gradient echo

Spin echo	Gradient echo
RF pulse is used to rephase	*Gradient* is applied to rephase
Uses flip angle of 90°	Uses variable flip angles
Slow sequence	Fast sequence

In conventional orthogonal planes in a spin echo sequence, the following can be derived:

- **Slice select:** At the same time as the 90° RF pulse is applied, DC current is sent to a separate RF coil to set a gradient along the z-axis for slice selection. The slice gradient is also switched on during the 180° pulse so that the rephasing pulse is specifically applied to the selected slice.
- **Phase encoding:** sets the gradient along the y-axis, usually just before the 180° RF pulse is applied.
- **Frequency encoding:** sets the gradient along the x-axis, during echo time.

Learning Points *(continued)*

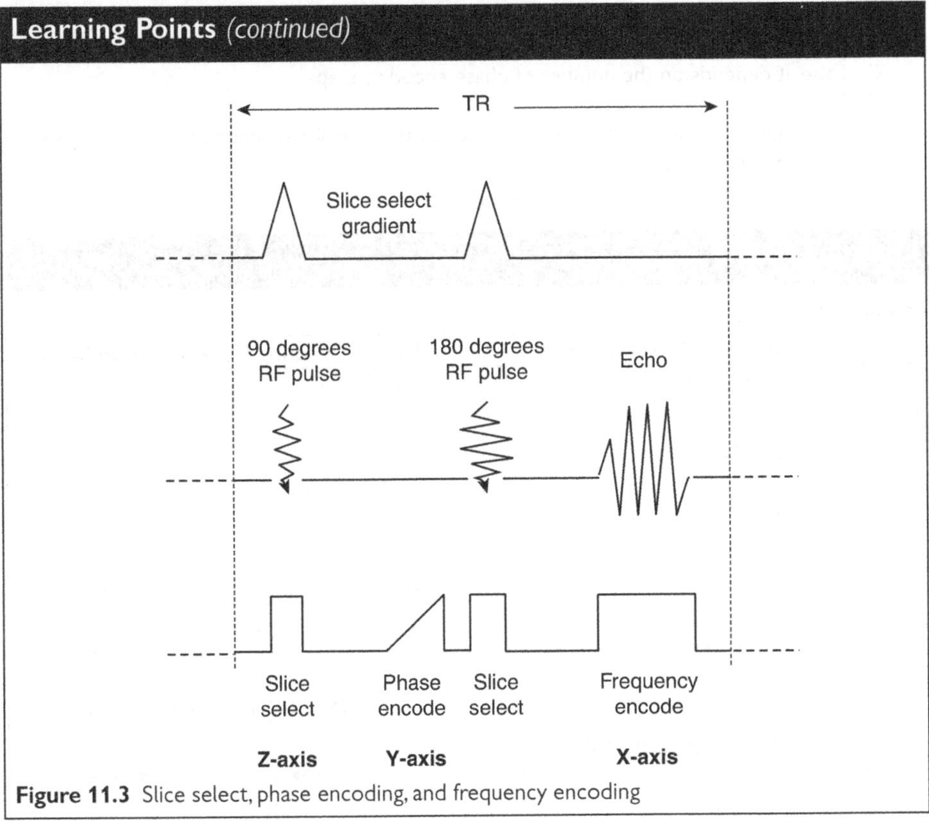

Figure 11.3 Slice select, phase encoding, and frequency encoding

19. A. True. This allows more longitudinal magnetization to recover with time.
B. False. Strictly speaking, using contrast increases contrast to noise ratio, and not SNR.
C. False. This is because by halving FOV (keeping the slice thickness the same), the voxel volume is reduced by a factor of 4. Therefore, although the spatial resolution is improved by a factor of 2, the SNR decreases more drastically by a factor of 4.
D. True. This increases the signal collected, although more noise is also sampled.
E. True. This increases voxel volume, and therefore SNR.

Westbrook. *Handbook of MRI Technique*, 3rd edn, Wiley-Blackwell, 2006. pp. 15–22.
Edelman, Hesselink, Zlatkin, & Crues. *Clinical Magnetic Resonance Imaging*, 3rd edn, Saunders Elsevier, 2005. pp. 90–96.

20. A. False. Increasing FOV increases voxel volume, therefore spatial resolution is reduced.
B. True. By increasing matrix size, the pixel, and therefore the voxel is smaller, improving spatial resolution.
C. True. This is because the voxel volume is increased.
D. True. Increasing frequency matrix increases resolution, without affecting scan time.
E. False. Using small coils improves SNR but does not directly affect spatial resolution.

Westbrook. *Handbook of MRI Technique*, 3rd edn, Wiley-Blackwell, 2006. pp. 15–22.

21. A. True. Scan time is = TR × number of phase encoding steps × NEX.
B. False.
C. False. It depends on the number of phase encoding steps.
D. True.
E. True. This is true in 3D-fast scan sequence as another phase encoding gradient is used to select and excite each slice.

Westbrook. *Handbook of MRI Technique*, 3rd edn, Wiley-Blackwell, 2006. pp. 18–19.

Learning Points

Table 11.3 Signal-to-noise ratio

Signal-to-Noise ratio is increased by	Factors affecting Signal-to-Noise Ratio
Scanning areas of high PD	Proton density
Increasing voxel volume	Field strength
Increasing TR and flip angle	Voxel size
Small and well positioned coils	Coil type and position
Increasing NEX	TR/TE
	Flip angle
Decreasing TE	Number of Signal Averages (NEX)
Decreasing receiving bandwidth	Receive bandwidth

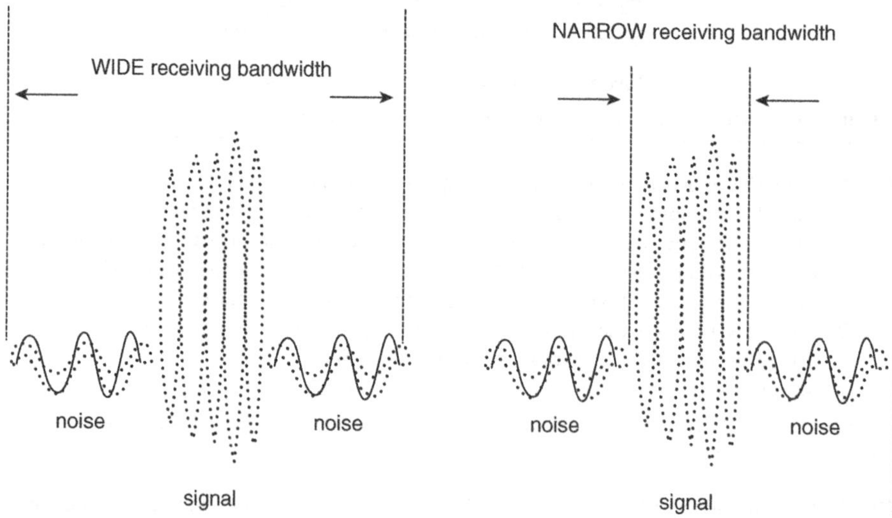

Figure 11.4 Wide and narrow receiving bandwidth

Figure 11.4 demonstrates how changing the receiving bandwidth affects signal-to-noise ratio. Reducing the receiving bandwidth reduces the amount of noise sampled and therefore increases the signal-to-noise ratio. The trade-off for doing this is that it increases the minimum TE and increases the effects of chemical shift artefact.

Learning Points *(continued)*

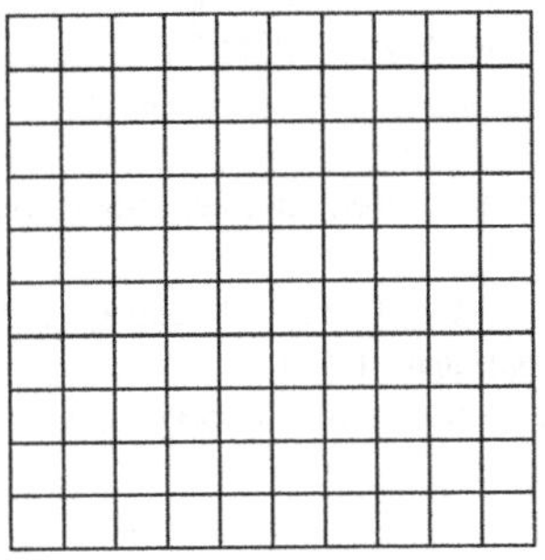

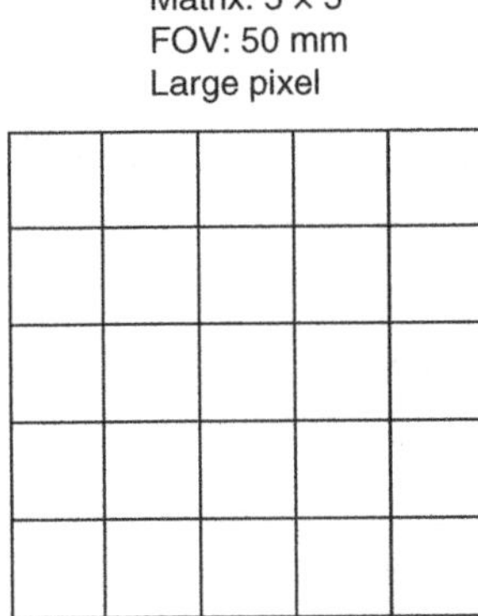

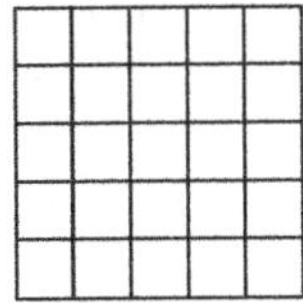

Figure 11.5 The difference between different matrix size and field of view (FOV)

Voxel Volume = field of view/matrix × slice thickness

Scan time = TR × number of phase encoding steps × NEX

Note that it depends on the phase encoding steps not the frequency encoding steps (NEX = number of signal averages).

22. A. True. The steeper the gradient, the smaller the FOV.
B. True.
C. False. See A.
D. True. This is usually 10–20ms.
E. False. Spatial information is not complete until all the gradient steps, usually 512 steps, are completed.

23. A. True.
B. False. This will make the effects more pronounced.
C. False. Decreasing the receiving bandwidth increases the likelihood of chemical shift artefact.
D. False. It manifests as an area of signal void. This is usually between areas of fat and water.
E. True. As this removes/suppresses fat signal.

Electronic Learning Database, E-Learning for Healthcare, Radiology—Integrated Training Initiative (R-ITI) – www.e-lfh.org.uk
Module: 8a_156: MRI Artefacts.
Zhuo & Gullapalli. 'AAPM/RSNA physics tutorial for residents: MR artifacts, safety, and quality control', *Radiographics*, Jan–Feb 2006; 26(1): 275–97. Review.

24. A. True.
B. False. It can be reduced by using a steeper gradient.
C. True.
D. False. The Dixon technique is used to combat chemical misregistration artefact.
E. True.

Westbrook. *Handbook of MRI Technique*, 3rd edn, Wiley-Blackwell, 2006. pp. 34–40.
Zhuo & Gullapalli. 'AAPM/RSNA physics tutorial for residents: MR artifacts, safety, and quality control', *Radiographics*, Jan–Feb 2006; 26(1): 275–97. Review.

25. A. False. In the frequency encoding axis.
B. True.
C. False. Often it occurs because the FOV is too small. Enlarging the FOV is often used to combat against this.
D. False. In the phase encoding direction.
E. True.

Westbrook. *Handbook of MRI Technique*, 3rd edn, Wiley-Blackwell, 2006. pp. 34–40.

26. A. True.
B. False. It shortens both T1 and T2 but the effect on T1 is greater.
C. True. Hence it is used with a chelating agent such as DTPA. Gd-DTPA is formed which can be safely excreted. Gd itself is extremely toxic.
D. True.
E. True.

Electronic Learning Database, E-Learning for Healthcare, Radiology—Integrated Training Initiative (R-ITI) – www.e-lfh.org.uk
Module: 8a_149: Contrast Agents.

27. A. False. It is a negative contrast agent and areas of uptake appear as low signal.
B. True. It is taken up by reticulo-endothelial system and excreted by liver. Normal liver tissue will appear as a low signal and liver lesions will appear as a high signal on T2-weighted images.
C. True.
D. False. It is known as a T2 enhancing agent.
E. True. Although, this is not used widely in normal clinical practice.

Westbrook. *Handbook of MRI Technique*, 3rd edn, Wiley-Blackwell, 2006. pp. 55–7.

28. A. True. MRI is contraindicated in patients with a pacemaker and they should be excluded from MR areas.
B. False. It is defined as areas where stray fields are greater than 0.5mT.
C. False. These are caused by alternating (time-varying) magnetic fields and not static magnetic fields. Other effects include light flashes, involuntary muscle contractions, and cardiac arrhythmias.
D. False. Hearing protection is required to prevent irreversible hearing damage.
E. True. The theoretical risk is due to excessive heating acting as a potential teratogen. Because of uncertainties in the RF dosimetry during pregnancy, it is recommended that exposure duration should be reduced to the minimum and that only the normal operation level is used, and to exclude pregnant women during the first three months of pregnancy.

Westbrook. *MRI at a Glance*, Blackwell Science, 2002. pp.96–100.
Shellock & Crues. 'MR procedures: biologic effects, safety, and patient care', *Radiology*, Sep 2004; 232(3): 635–52.

29. A. True. SAR depends on induced electric field, pulse duty cycle, tissue density, conductivity, and the patient's size. In the UK, it is recommended that temperature should not exceed 1°C during an examination.
B. True.
C. True.
D. True.
E. True.

Refer to the latest Medicines and Healthcare products and Regulatory Agency (MHRA)'s Safety Guidelines for Magnetic Resonance Imaging Equipment in Clinical Use, Dec 2007 http://www.mhra.gov.uk

30. A. False. It results in several days downtime.
B. False. It may result in severe and irreparable damage and is done only in an emergency situation.
C. False. Following quenching, helium escapes into the environment and the room should be vented to remove helium to the outside. In a closed room, helium will replace oxygen and increases pressure in a closed room. As accidental quenching can occur without the operator's knowledge, a room must be fitted with an oxygen monitor which will sound an alarm if oxygen level falls below a threshold.
D. False. The patient should be transferred to an MR-compatible trolley and then be taken outside the control area where the arrest team can take over.
E. False. Fire fighting equipment should be used only at a safe distance which depends on field gradient, strength, and active shielding. Ideally, only carbon dioxide extinguishers should be used. Quenching should occur if firemen need to enter inner controlled areas. As a general rule, it is not advisable to take non-MRI safe equipment into the scan room.

Westbrook. *MRI at a Glance*, Blackwell Science, 2002. pp.96–100.
Shellock & Crues. 'MR procedures: biologic effects, safety, and patient care', *Radiology*, Sep 2004; 232(3): 635–52.

31. A. True.
B. False. Only up to about 0.3T.
C. True.
D. False. Absolute zero is currently unachievable, but they are cooled to 4 degrees Kelvin and at this temperature there is negligible resistance.
E. False. A Faraday cage is used to shield the scanner from external RF interference.

Westbrook. *MRI at a Glance*, Blackwell Science, 2002. pp.90–5.
Edelman, Hesselink, Zlatkin, & Crues. *Clinical Magnetic Resonance Imaging*, 3rd edn, Saunders Elsevier, 2005. pp. 109–29.

32. A. True.
B. False. 10ppm is required.
C. True. Usually, 1ppm is required.
D. False. Stray fringe fields are significant for both resistive and superconductive electromagnets.
E. False. See D.

Westbrook. *MRI at a Glance*, Blackwell Science, 2002. pp.90–5.
Edelman, Hesselink, Zlatkin, & Crues. *Clinical Magnetic Resonance Imaging*, 3rd edn, Saunders Elsevier, 2005. pp. 109–29.

33. A. False. Loud banging noises are caused by switching off the currents in the gradient coils.
B. True.
C. True.
D. True.
E. False. Surface or local receiver coils are separate coils to the main scanner and are applied as closely to the patient's body part of interest as possible. This is to allow for better resolution.

Westbrook. *MRI at a Glance*, Blackwell Science, 2002. pp.90–5.
Edelman, Hesselink, Zlatkin, & Crues. *Clinical Magnetic Resonance Imaging*, 3rd edn, Saunders Elsevier, 2005. pp. 109–29.

34. A. False. The recommendation is that staff should not be exposed to more than 2T for the whole body and 5T for limbs. These are the basic restrictions for occupational exposure to static magnetic fields.
B. True.
C. True.
D. False. The extent and steepness of the fringe field gradient depends on the main magnet field strength, the design of magnet (open versus tunnel bore) and the shielding employed (active, passive cladding, or whole room shielding). Each installation will differ due to the surrounding structures and therefore it is essential that staff at every MR site should have a thorough understanding of the fringe fields relating to each scanner that is on their site.
E. True. A field strength of 0.5mT (5 Gauss) was chosen for the MR CONTROLLED AREA to avoid interaction with medical implants. A field strength of 3mT (30 Gauss) was chosen for the INNER MR CONTROLLED AREA to avoid the projectile hazard.

Health Protection Agency (HPA) Publications (www.hpa.org.uk):
MRI - EC Physical Agents Directive (4 September 2008)
Static Magnetic Fields (RCE-6) (1 September 2008)
Electronic Learning Database, E-Learning for Healthcare, Radiology—Integrated Training Initiative (R-ITI) – www.e-lfh.org.uk
Module: 8a_144: Metal and MR Safety.

35. A. True.
B. True. Time-varying magnetic fields induce electric currents that potentially interfere with the normal function of nerve cells and muscle fibres. An example of this is peripheral nerve stimulation (PNS). A more serious response to electric currents flowing through the body is that of ventricular fibrillation, which is prevented in clinical scanners operating within International Electrotechnical Commission (IEC) limits.
C. True.
D. True. One fundamental issue is excessive cardiovascular strain resulting from thermoregulatory responses to body temperatures raised over a short period of time by more than 0.5°C in vulnerable people. MR scanners limit temperature rise by limiting SAR.
E. True.

National Radiological Protection Board. *ELF electromagnetic fields and the risk of cancer; report of an advisory group on non-ionising radiation.* Documents of the NRPB 12(1), 2001. ISBN 0859514560. http://www.hpa.org.uk/radiation/publications/documents_of_nrpb/abstracts/absd12-1.htm.

36. A. True.
B. True.
C. True.
D. True.
E. True. All are important considerations in QA and methods used to acquire these are beyond the scope of this book, are likely to vary from different institutions and also depend on the manufacture of individual scanners.

Firbank et al. 'Quality assurance for MRI: practical experience', *The British Journal of Radiology*, 2000; 73(868): pp. 376–83.

37. A. False. 'Moving blood' appears as low signal on SE.
B. True.
C. True.
D. True.
E. False. Short T1 tissues such as fat can leave a residual signal in ToF angiography and can obscure the anatomy of blood vessels and therefore must be interpreted accordingly.

Electronic Learning Database, E-Learning for Healthcare, Radiology—Integrated Training Initiative (R-ITI) – www.e-lfh.org.uk
Module: 8a_152: Magnetic Resonance Angiography (MRA).

38. A. True. Although it is not specific to it, i.e. fat, methaemoglobin, melanin, lesions enhanced by gadolinium.
B. True.
C. False. Apparent diffusion coefficient (ADC) is also required in conjunction for interpretation.
D. False. FLAIR is used to null a signal from fluid. For example, it can be used in brain imaging to suppress cerebrospinal fluid (CSF) so as to demonstrate hyperintense lesions, such as multiple sclerosis (MS) plaques.
E. True.

Westbrook. *Handbook of MRI Technique*, 3rd edn, Wiley-Blackwell, 2006. pp. 22–33.

39. A. False. This would be less than ideal as STIR suppresses short T1 tissues (which includes Gd-DTPA enhanced tissues).
B. True.
C. True.
D. True.
E. False. Melanin appears as high signal on T1.

40. A. True.
B. True.
C. True. They consist of STIR type fat signal suppression (inversion-recovery), and suppression of the water signal by selective saturation pulse centred on its resonance frequency peak. This enables the differentiation of silicone (which is also a high signal on T2) and water. This is particularly useful to detect implant rupture.
D. True. Manganese chelates are known as hepato-biliary contrast agents and normal tissues that take up contrast will display a high signal on T1.
E. True. This is to cope with the constraints of temporal resolution and T2* sensitivity.

Edelman, Hesselink, Zlatkin, & Crues. *Clinical Magnetic Resonance Imaging*, 3rd edn, Saunders Elsevier, 2005. p. 97.

APPENDIX: USEFUL EQUATIONS

$c = \lambda f$

$E = hc/\lambda = hf$

c = speed of light (299 800km/s)
λ = wavelength
f = frequency of radiation
E = Energy
h = Planck's constant (4.13×10^{-18} keV/s)

Photoelectric effects:
No of interactions $\alpha \quad Z^3.\rho/E^3$

Z = atomic number
ρ = density of material

Compton scatter:
No of interactions $\alpha \ \rho/E$
Wavelength change $\Delta\lambda = 0.0024(1-\cos\Phi)$
(i.e. wavelength change is dependent on angle of scatter)

X-rays Generation:

$$\text{Quantity } \alpha \ \frac{Z.\,\text{mAs}\,.\,\text{kV}^2\,.\,\rho^2\,.\,\text{waveform}}{d^2\,.\,\text{filtration}\,.\,2^{\,\text{nHVL}}}$$

nHVL = no of Half Value Layer

Quality α kV . waveform . filtration

Linear attenuation coefficient (LAC) = μ *[unit = mm^{-1}]*

$\mu_{total} = \Sigma\,[\mu_{elastic} + \mu_{Compton} + \mu_{photoelectric}]$
Total attenuation = product of each attenuating process

$$\mu = \frac{0.693}{HVL}$$

Mass attenuation coefficient (MAC) *[unit = cm^2/g]*

$$MAC = \frac{LAC}{\rho}$$

Tube rating:

$$\text{Tube rating } \alpha \ \frac{\text{(effective) focal spot size . anode speed . waveform}}{\text{exposure time . kV . target } \theta}$$

Focal spot size:

$$\text{Effective focal spot size } \alpha \ \frac{\text{filament size . anode angle } \theta \text{ . mA}}{\text{kVp}}$$

Grid:

$$\text{Grid Factor} = \frac{\text{Exposure with grid}}{\text{Exposure without grid}}$$

Intensifying Screens:

$$\text{Intensification Factor} = \frac{\text{Exposure without screen}}{\text{Exposure with screen}}$$

$$\text{Intensification Factor} \ \alpha \ \frac{\text{kV . Thickness . size}}{\text{Dose}}$$

Contrast:

Subject contrast α subject thickness . density . atomic Z . kV

Unsharpness:

Total unsharpness (U_t) is the square root of the sum of individually squared components

$$U_t = \sqrt{U_g^2 + U_p^2 + U_m^2 + U_a^2}$$

Magnification:

$$\text{Mag} = \frac{\text{FFD}}{\text{FOD}}$$

FFD = Field to Focus distance
FOD = Field to Object distance

Modulation Transfer Function (MTF):

$$\text{MTF} = \frac{\text{output modulation}}{\text{Input}}$$

MTF of system = Σ [MTF_1 to MTF_n]

$$\text{MTF} \ \alpha \ \frac{\text{magnification}}{\text{FOD . spatial freq}}$$

Image Intensifier

$$\text{Brightness Gain (Intensification Factor)} = \frac{\text{Brightness of output phosphur}}{\text{Brightness of input phosphur}}$$

= Minification gain × Flux gain

Minification Gain = (Øinput / Øoutput)^2

$$\text{Conversion efficiency} = \frac{\text{Luminance of output phosphor}}{\text{Input exposure rate}}$$

Computed Tomography:

CT Dose Index (CTDI):

$$\text{CTDI} = \frac{\text{Area under the curve}}{\text{Slice thickness (T)}} = \frac{\int D(z)\,.\,dz}{T}$$

$$CTDI_{weighted} = 1/3\ CTDI_{centre} + 2/3\ CTDI_{periphery}$$

$$CTDI_{volume} = CTDI_{weighted} / \text{pitch}$$

Dose Length Product (DLP)

DLP = $CTDI_{vol} \times L = CTDI_w$. length / pitch

Length = no of rotations . collimated length . pitch

CT Dose

CT Dose α $\frac{\text{mAs . kV}}{\text{pitch}}$ α rotation time α resolution^3

$$\text{Pitch} = \frac{\text{Table excursion (mm/s) . gantry rotation time (s)}}{\text{collimation (mm)}}$$

Ultrasound:

Length of near field $= a^2/\lambda$ — a = transducer radius

Far field divergence $\sin\theta = 0.61\lambda/a$

Doppler shift frequency $(f_d) = f_t - f_r = 2 f_t v \cos\theta / c$

- f_t = Transmitted frequency
- f_r = Received frequency
- v = Velocity of reflector
- c = Speed of sound in medium
- θ = Angle between the beam and moving object

Acoustic impedance $(z) = \rho.c$

$c^2 = k / \rho$

- ρ = density of material
- k = stiffness/incompressibility

Lateral resolution α f/a

Axial resolution α f/pulse length

Magnetic resonance:

$\omega = \gamma.\beta_0$

- ω = precessional frequency
- γ = gyromagnetic ratio
- β_0 = external magnetic field

INDEX

Key: ■ denotes question, ■ denotes answer